Cover designed by Dimart Studio (www.dimart-studio.com)

Designed by Claire Guigal (www.claireguigal.com)

Edited by Ann C. Moller (www.annmollerthemuse.com)

Published by Oculus Publishers, Inc. (www.oculuspublishers.com)

THE YEAR ONE CHALLENGE FOR WOMEN
THINNER, LEANER, AND STRONGER THAN EVER IN 12 MONTHS

BY MICHAEL MATTHEWS

To everyone who has supported and believed in me,
including my readers, followers, parents, wife, friends, and colleagues.

I probably don't thank you all often enough,
but I really do mean it when I do.

PRAISE FOR THINNER LEANER STRONGER

"If you want to use strength training for aesthetics, Mike is your source. Read this book, and read mine too, and come away with what you need to know. The rest will be up to you."

—Mark Rippetoe, author of *Starting Strength: Basic Barbell Training and Practical Programming for Strength Training*

"Nobody cuts through the fitness and nutrition confusion and clutter like Mike Matthews. And in *Thinner Leaner Stronger*, he draws on a powerful combination of time in the trenches and hard-core research to give you the straight talk about what actually works.

"This book is easy to read and incredibly effective. I highly recommend."

—Ben Greenfield, CEO of Kion & New York Times bestselling author of *Beyond Training: Mastering Endurance, Health & Life*

"Mike has written the encyclopedia of body recomposition for the twentieth century. A great book and a must-buy for beginners looking to get their feet wet."

—Martin Berkhan, fitness coach, pioneer, and author of *The Leangains Method*

"Mike Matthews stands alone in the fitness space. His books are based on scientific research and real-world results. *Thinner Leaner Stronger* can change your life."

—Strauss Zelnick, "America's fittest CEO" and author of *Becoming Ageless: The Four Secrets to Looking and Feeling Younger Than Ever*

"In *Thinner Leaner Stronger*, Mike takes us back to the fundamentals of losing fat and building muscle—time-tested and science-backed strategies that have been obscured by a rising tide of popular hype and pseudoscience.

"The good news: it doesn't have to be that hard!"

—Alex Hutchinson, author of the New York Times bestseller *Endure: Mind, Body, and the Curiously Elastic Limits of Human Performance*

"Matthews has masterfully distilled many years of research into the essence of what makes people fit—and fast.

"His training methods have worked better than anything else I've tried for improving my strength and physique. Get this book right now."

—Stephen Guise, international bestselling author of *Mini Habits*

"Mike Matthews has done it again. Great information backed by science, and complicated knowledge transformed into practical, applicable strategies.

"I loved *Thinner Leaner Stronger*. A must-read."

—Adam Schafer, co-host of top-ranked fitness and health podcast *Mind Pump*

"I haven't been this excited to about a fitness book in years. It's required reading for all gals who want to get—and stay—in the best shape of their lives. A true classic in the making."

—Sal Di Stefano, co-host of top-ranked fitness and health podcast *Mind Pump*

"Would you rather spend a month of your life hoping the latest flavor of diet and exercise plan will work . . . or spend thirty days knowing your hard work will provide results you can not only see, but feel?

"Give me guaranteed results any day, and that's what *Thinner Leaner Stronger* provides—all the knowledge and motivation you need to get results for years to come."

—Jeff Haden, Inc. Magazine contributing editor and author of *The Motivation Myth: How High Achievers Really Set Themselves Up to Win*

"*Thinner Leaner Stronger* gives you everything you need to know for achieving the body you want. Full stop. No hype and no gimmicks, just solid info backed by solid science. An outstanding book."

—James Krieger, MS, founder of *Weightology* (www.weightology.net)

"As a clinical practitioner who specializes in obesity medicine, I truly appreciate *Thinner Leaner Stronger*. It's simple, science-based, and most importantly, it works, and that's why I recommend it to many of my patients.

"Drop whatever you're doing and read this book. It can change your life."

—Dr. Spencer Nadolsky, board-certified family and obesity medicine physician and founder of RP Health

"A highly actionable book that translates the latest science into a simple plan for strength. In a world filled with noise, Mike Matthews provides the clarity and practical strategies you need to get results."

—James Clear, author of *Atomic Habits: An Easy & Proven Way to Build Good Habits & Break Bad Ones*

FREE BONUS MATERIAL (VIDEOS, TOOLS, AND MORE!)

Thank you for choosing *The Year One Challenge for Women*.

I hope you find it insightful, inspiring, and practical, and I hope it helps you build that lean, sculpted, and strong body you really desire.

I want to make sure that you get as much value from this program as possible, so I've put together a number of additional free resources to help you, including:

→ All of the workouts neatly laid out and provided in several formats, including PDF, Excel, and Google Sheets.

→ Links to form demonstration videos for all *Thinner Leaner Stronger* exercises.

→ 10 *Thinner Leaner Stronger* meal plans that make losing fat and gaining lean muscle as simple as possible.

→ A Google Sheets meal planning template for simpler and easier meal planning.

→ A list of my favorite tools for getting and staying motivated and on track inside and outside of the gym.

→ And more.

To get instant access to all of those free bonuses (plus a few additional surprise gifts), go here now:

→ www.thinnerleanerstronger.com/challengebonus

Also, if you have any questions or run into any difficulties, just shoot me an e-mail at mike@muscleforlife.com and I'll do my best to help!

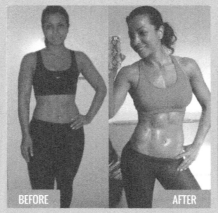

*"I liked that it gave me direction
and motivation every time
I went to the gym"*

YVONNE A.

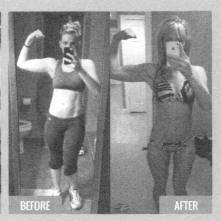

*"I lost 10 pounds and gained
of muscle in 7 months!"*

MARSHA M.

*"It was the perfect book to educate
and guide me."*

CHRISSIE R.

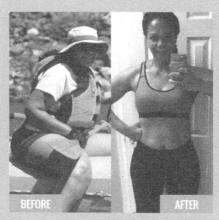

*"I have more energy,
discipline, and have gained
more confidence!"*

SUSIE G.

*"I am happier about myself, more
confident, and I get compliments about
my fitness which makes me smile!"*

LOUISE C.

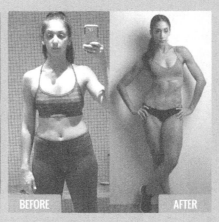

*"Eating the correct balance
of macros has given me
more consistent energy and
I no longer have crashes."*

KATHY V.

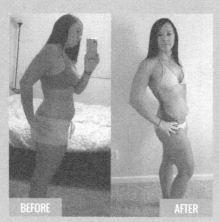

*"I never expected that
I'd be able to get as fit
and healthy as I am today."*

ALI P

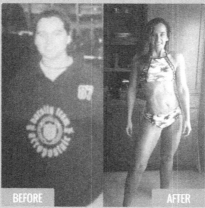

*"I have more energy and
confidence, and as a whole am a
completely different person."*

JILL A.

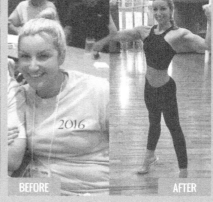

*"For the first time in my life, I feel
comfortable in my own skin."*

ALICE S.

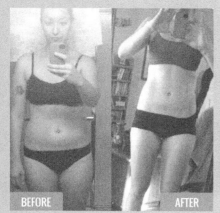

"I think I could write a book about how this program has changed my life."

ALEXIS E.

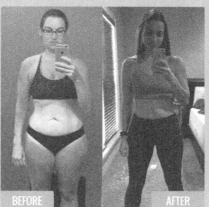

"It sounds cliche, but this has honestly changed my life. I have become happier and a better mother to my children."

RACHEL M.

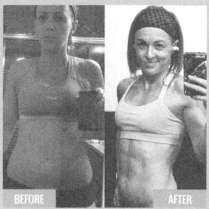

"This book helped me take control of my life. Trust the process and just keep going."

LIZ T.

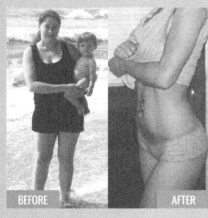

"I lost 50 lbs in 7 months following Mike's books!"

KELLY O.

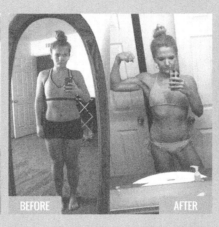

"I have never truly been this healthy in my life. I feel strong and sexy and finally have the confidence I have always wanted."

SHAY B.

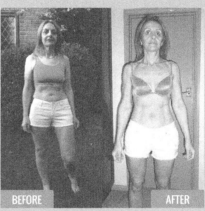

"I've lost 8 kg (17 lbs) so far!"

LAURA M.

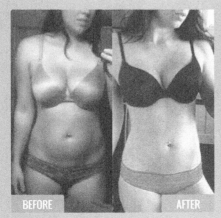

"I'm a beast. I lost 23 pounds and feel like a solid human made of meat no fat."

TARA Z.

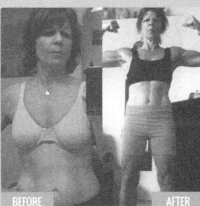

"I feel younger, more energetic, and happy!"

ANGELA A.

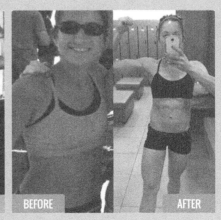

"It's so amazing how my body has transformed in the last few weeks!"

KATIE T.

IT WORKS! ORDINARY WOMEN, EXTRAORDINARY RESULTS. WILL YOU BE NEXT?

The women you just saw are just like you.

They're in their 30s, 40s, and 50s, and they come from all walks of life and levels of fitness. Some were once fit, others were always overweight, some had tried many diet and exercise routines before and failed, others were brand new to it all, some had a lot of time and energy for working out, and others had very little.

What they all have in common, though, is they've all used the diet and exercise principles and programs you're about to learn to get into the best shape of their lives.

Every one of these women has dropped pounds of unwanted fat, added lean muscle in all the right places, and dramatically reduced their risk of disease and dysfunction.

And they did it eating the foods they love, doing workouts they enjoy, and taking few, if any, supplements.

I want to introduce you to several of them whose stories have inspired and touched me, and who are definitive proof that with the right know-how and guidance, anyone can build a body they can be proud of.

If they can do it, why not you?

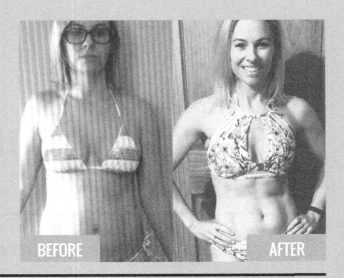

BEFORE   AFTER

AMBER'S STORY

I really never struggled with weight until after my third baby. In the two years after she was born, I ran a half marathon and I did other weightlifting programs to no avail.

I was completely defeated and almost resigned to the fact that maybe it was just my age or stage of life.

When I couldn't drop the weight, I felt terrible about myself. I was constantly beating myself up because I had never struggled the way I was struggling.

Then I started the *Thinner Leaner Stronger* program, and I was shocked at how quickly the weight started to fall off. Results were quick for me because I started being honest with myself about what I was eating and not doing.

After starting the program, I dieted for eight weeks and lost 14 pounds, and I haven't gained any weight for a year.

I'm most proud of the amount of weight I can lift. I'm a little person by bone structure, but I feel SO STRONG! My squat increased by 45 pounds, my deadlift increased by 65 pounds, and my leg press increased by 110 pounds!

This program is superior to any program out there. It wasn't just about dropping weight, either—it was about taking time for myself as a mom and finding just one way to put myself first.

I'm most proud of my strength and that my kids ask me to flex on the daily—especially my girls.

Ninety-nine percent of the time after my workouts, I'm happy, energized, and ready to conquer my two jobs, kids, home life, and everything else on my plate.

The thing I've repeated to myself over and over is "trust the process." I trust Mike Matthews and his no-nonsense, "this is science" approach. Read the book, apply it, and you WILL see results.

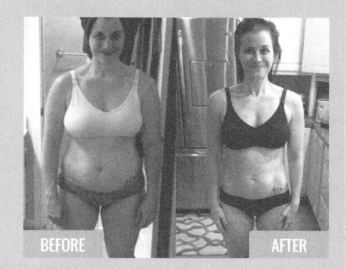

BEFORE   AFTER

JENNA'S STORY

I was sick of spending hours in the gym doing CARDIO, CARDIO, CARDIO and not getting result. It worked okay for me when I was younger, but after having several children along with getting older, it just wasn't working, and I felt stuck at a certain number on the scale.

Since starting *Thinner Leaner Stronger*, I've lost 35 pounds in six months! I've also noticed that my energy levels have increased, my mood is better, and I don't fight unhealthy cravings the way I used to.

Overall, I just feel so much better.

I increased my bench press by 40 pounds, my squat by 60 pounds, my deadlift by 45 pounds, and my leg press by 240 pounds. In the past I would just do cycling, running, or elliptical—I had never lifted weights before. I relied mainly on counting calories and cardio to stay at my ideal weight.

This program is truly a lifestyle and is completely sustainable. I'm not quite at the maintenance stage yet, but I know it'll be even more flexible once I get to that point.

I have so much more to learn and new goals to set, but I'm genuinely enjoying the process. I really appreciate the self-discipline this program has taught me.

By following *Thinner Leaner Stronger*, you're building the body you want for the rest of your life, and it takes time, consistency, and patience. But it's worth it. Watching your body change is an amazing thing and very empowering.

I've managed to follow this program faithfully with three children under the age of four—one who is seven months old and exclusively breastfed. If I can do it under these circumstances, anyone can do it!

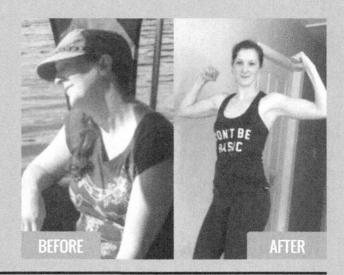

BEFORE AFTER

GENEVIEVE'S STORY

My friend and long-distance fitness coach told me that if I followed the *Thinner Leaner Stronger* program, I'd be extremely happy with the results.

He said it wasn't complicated but that I had to have the motivation and willingness to work hard. He was right.

In one year and nine months, I lost 34 pounds and 8 percent body fat. I also added 55 pounds to my deadlift, 45 pounds to my squat, and got my bench press up to 50 pounds!

It took me some time to get into the rhythm of things. Once I realized how badly I wanted to lose weight and gain core strength, I noticed my body changing fast. (After having two children, my core strength was nonexistent.)

I saw results immediately, and that made me push harder to achieve my goals and make new ones.

When it comes to the workouts, the heavy weightlifting made me feel good, and I liked how Mike broke down proper form for every exercise. On the nutrition side of things, once I calculated a few breakfast, lunch, and dinner options, it wasn't so hard.

I'm definitely more confident now, too. I'm able to show my daughters that staying healthy and being strong is important in more ways than one. I have more energy, which is great for work, and I'm able to keep up with my kids after work.

I even had the courage to sign up for a Spartan Race this summer!

I'd recommend *Thinner Leaner Stronger* to anyone who's skeptical about working out. I've never been a gym person, and Mike Matthews made it accessible and fun for me.

Read the book, then reread it and take notes. Create a list of simple goals you'd like to achieve. Then set more goals once you've achieved those.

I hope you enjoyed those success stories as much as I did...

... and are inspired to follow in the footsteps of the outstanding women you just met.

Who knows, maybe people will be reading about your transformation story one day?

Anything is possible if you want it enough.
And in this book, I'm going to show you the way.

WHO IS MIKE MATTHEWS AND WHY SHOULD I CARE?

Opportunity is missed by most people,
because it is dressed in overalls and looks like work.

—UNKNOWN

I'm Mike, and I believe that every person can achieve the body of their dreams.

My mission is to give everyone that opportunity by providing time-proven, evidence-based advice on how to build muscle, lose fat, and get and stay healthy.

I've been training for more than a decade now. In that time, I've read thousands of pages of scientific literature and tried just about every type of workout program, diet regimen, and supplement you can imagine. At this point, I can confidently say that while I don't know everything, I do know what works and what doesn't.

Like most people who get into weightlifting, I had no clue what I was doing when I started out. I turned to fitness magazines for help, which told me to spend a couple of hours in the gym every day and hundreds of dollars on pills and powders every month. This went on for years, and I jumped from diet to diet, workout program to workout program, and supplement to supplement, only to make mediocre progress and eventually get stuck in a rut.

I then turned to personal trainers for guidance, but they had me do more of the same. After spending many thousands of dollars with them, I still hadn't gained any more muscle or strength to speak of, and I still had no idea what to do with my diet and training to reach my goals. I liked working out too much to quit, but I wasn't happy with my body and didn't know what I was doing wrong.

I finally decided that something had to change, and I knew that I needed to start with learning the actual physiology of muscle growth and fat loss. So I threw the magazines away, fired the trainers, got off the internet forums, and instead began searching out the work of top strength and bodybuilding coaches, talking to scores of natural bodybuilders, and reading scientific papers.

Several months later, a clear picture was beginning to emerge.

The real science of getting into incredible shape is very simple—much simpler than the fitness industry wants us to believe. It flies in the face of a lot of the stuff we see on TV, Instagram, and YouTube and read in books, articles, and magazines.

For example . . .

→ You don't need supplements to build a great physique.

→ You don't need to constantly change up your workout routine to "confuse" your muscles.

→ You don't need to "eat clean" to get and stay lean.

→ You don't need to stop eating carbs and sugars to lose weight.

→ You don't need to eat small meals every few hours to "boost your metabolism."

→ You don't need to grind out hours and hours of boring cardio every week to get a ripped core.

→ You don't need to be in the gym hours per day and sacrifice your relationships with your friends and loved ones.

As a result of what I had learned, I completely changed my approach to eating and exercising, and my body responded in ways I couldn't believe. My strength skyrocketed. My muscles started growing again. My energy levels went through the roof. And here's the kicker: I was spending less time in the gym, doing less cardio, and eating foods I actually liked.

Along the way, my friends and family noticed how my physique was improving and began asking for advice. I became their coach. I took "hardgainers" and put 30 pounds on them in a year, took people who were absolutely baffled as to why they couldn't lose weight and stripped away piles of fat, and took people in their 40s, 50s, and 60s who believed their hormones and metabolisms were beyond repair and helped them get into the best shape of their lives.

A couple of years later, these people started urging me to write a book. I dismissed the idea at first, but eventually I began to warm up to it. "What if I'd had such a book when I started training?" I thought. It would have saved me who knows how much time, money, and frustration, and I would have built the body of my dreams a lot faster. I also enjoyed helping people with what I had learned, and if I were to write a book and it became popular, what if I could help thousands or even hundreds of thousands of people?

That gave me a wild hair, and so I wrote *Bigger Leaner Stronger* and published it in January 2012. It sold maybe 20 copies in the first month, but within a couple of months, sales were growing, and I began receiving emails from readers with high praise. I was ecstatic. I started making notes on how I could improve the book based on feedback, and I outlined ideas for several other books that I could write.

Fast-forward to today, and I've now published a number of books, including a companion book (*Thinner Leaner Stronger*), and a "flexible dieting" cookbook (*The Shredded Chef*). Altogether, my books have sold over a million copies, and my work has been featured in a number of publications like *Women's Health, Muscle & Strength, Elle, Esquire*, and more.

More importantly, every day I get scores of emails and social media messages from readers who are thankful for my work and blown away by the results they're seeing. They're just as shocked as I was years ago when I first discovered just how straightforward and enjoyable getting fit and healthy can really be.

This is why I continue to write books and articles, record podcasts and YouTube videos, and generally do everything I can to be as helpful to as many people as I can. It's motivating to see the impact I'm having on people's lives, and I'm incredibly inspired by the dedication and determination of so many of my readers and followers. You guys and gals rock.

I also have bigger ambitions that I want to realize.

First, I want to help a million people get fit and healthy. "Help a million people" just has a sexy ring to it, don't you think? It's a big goal, but I think I can do it.

This goes beyond merely making people look hotter.

I want to make a dent in some of the alarming downward trends we're seeing here in the Western world—in particular, the decline of people's physical and mental health and performance, which has significant and negative downstream effects in their family lives, careers, and personal happiness and satisfaction. I think helping people get strong and fit is a great way to do something about this.

Second, I want to lead the fight against mainstream health and fitness pseudoscience and BS.

Unfortunately, this space is full of misinformation, disinformation, idiots, liars, and hucksters, and I want to help change the status quo. I'd like to become known as the go-to guy for practical, easy-to-understand advice grounded in real science and results.

Third, I want to help reform the sport supplements industry.

The pill and powder pushers use all types of scams to foist their junk products on unwitting consumers. They use fancy-sounding-but-worthless ingredients; they cut their products with junk fillers like flour and useless amino acids; they use tiny, ineffective doses of otherwise good ingredients ("pixie dusting") and hide it with the notorious "proprietary blend"; and they rely on fake science, overhyped marketing claims, and steroid-fueled meatheads to convince people they have the "secret sauce."

So, that's me. From this point on, it's all going to be about you.

I hope you enjoy this book, and I hope it helps you reach your health and fitness goals faster.

Mike Matthews,
Vienna, Virginia, August 3, 2018

———————

P.S. If you're on social media, come say hi! Here's where you can find me:
Facebook: www.facebook.com/muscleforlifefitness
Instagram: www.instagram.com/muscleforlifefitness
YouTube: www.youtube.com/muscleforlifefitness
Twitter: www.twitter.com/muscleforlife

WELCOME TO THE YEAR ONE CHALLENGE FOR WOMEN

Make the most of yourself by fanning the tiny, inner sparks of possibility into flames of achievement.

—GOLDA MEIR

Welcome to the *Year One Challenge for Women*!

I'm incredibly excited that you're here because it means you've probably read my book *Thinner Leaner Stronger* and are ready to start the program.

(If you haven't read *Thinner Leaner Stronger* yet, you may want to do that first because this challenge assumes that you understand the training principles, strategies, and techniques taught in that book.)

I bet you're excited, too, because you have a huge year of personal transformation ahead of you, both inside and outside of the gym. I created this challenge and journal to help you make that happen in the biggest and best possible way.

As you've probably guessed, the Year One Challenge consists of a year's worth of *Thinner Leaner Stronger* workouts—six training phases in all—designed by me. In other words, this is exactly what I would have you do for the first year if I were personally training you.

These workouts are going to be fun, challenging, and most importantly, effective. They're also going to familiarize you with all of the key exercises you learned about in *Thinner Leaner Stronger*, so you can see firsthand which ones your body responds to best.

This way, when you start creating your own workout routines, you'll have all the experience you need to create workouts that will continue to produce results and that you'll also enjoy doing.

HOW TO USE THIS JOURNAL

This journal contains six training phases of workouts for the five-, four-, and three-day *Thinner Leaner Stronger* routines, including deload weeks and instructions for tracking your progress as you move through the program.

As you've learned, each phase of *Thinner Leaner Stronger* is comprised of eight weeks of hard training followed by one week of deloading and taking body measurements.

As far as results go, the five-day routine is better than the four- and three-day routines, and the four-day routine is better than the three-day routine. That doesn't mean you can't see great results with both the three- and four-day routines, though, because you can.

Try not to change routines during individual training phases. Ideally, you'd choose one routine and stick with it for the entire phase. That said, if you'd like to increase to the four- or five-day routine in the middle of a phase, go for it. Try not to "downgrade" unless you have to.

If you have the time and inclination, start with the five-day routine in your first training phase and see how you like it. You can always try the other routines in later phases.

Most people who follow the five-day routine train Monday through Friday and take the weekends off, but you can work in your rest days however you'd like. The important thing is you do each of the workouts every seven days and in the order given.

One caveat, however, is that you'll want to include at least one day of rest in between workouts 5 and 1, as doing these workouts on back-to-back days would be counterproductive.

So, for example, if you need to train on the weekends due to your schedule or lifestyle, you might train Monday (lower body), Tuesday (push and core), and Wednesday (pull), rest Thursday, then train Friday (upper body and core) and Saturday (lower body), and rest Sunday.

The workouts are laid out in simple charts that list the exercises and hard sets you're supposed to do in each. There's no space for recording warm-up sets because you don't need to track these. Do the exercises in the order given and fill in each hard set as you complete it, writing the weight followed by the reps.

You'll also notice that some exercises are bolded and italicized. This indicates you should do warm-up sets before your hard sets.

In the "notes" sections, you can record details about how your workout went as well as keep tabs on key factors that influence performance like diet, sleep, and general stress levels. For instance, you might note down that you slept well the night before and felt particularly strong in today's workout, or that you were short on calories the day before and noticed a slight decrease in energy during your training.

Here's an example of how a completed workout might look:

EXERCICES			
LOWER BODY			
Barbell Squat	135 × 9	135 × 9	135 × 8
Leg Press	155 × 10	165 × 8	165 × 8
Romanian Deadlift	105 × 9	105 × 8	105 × 7
Hip Thrust	135 × 10	145 × 8	145 × 8

NOTES: Felt very focused and strong today. Hamstring cramped during third set of Romanian deadlifts so had to bail a rep early.

DO YOU WANT ONE-ON-ONE COACHING?

If you'd like personal, hands-on help implementing everything you've learned in *Thinner Leaner Stronger*, including custom diet, exercise, and supplementation plans, then you need to check out my VIP one-on-one coaching service.

In just a few short years, we've worked with over 450 men and women all around the world and helped them do a lot more than lose a bunch of fat and gain a bunch of strength and muscle.

→ We've helped them skyrocket their grades and productivity.

→ We've helped them rekindle their love lives and even save their marriages.

→ We've helped them break food, drug, and alcohol addictions.

→ We've helped them form deeper bonds with friends and family.

→ We've helped them reverse and resolve health conditions and ditch medications.

And so much more . . .

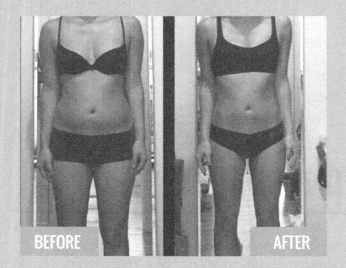

BEFORE   **AFTER**

ESTHER H.

For example, Esther (30) shows what you can accomplish when experts do all the thinking for you and make your dieting and training paint-by-numbers simple.

As you can see, she dramatically improved her body composition, but she also gained a tremendous amount of strength. For instance, when she started with us, she was deadlifting just the bar, and by the end of her 90-day coaching experience, she was close to her body weight for reps.

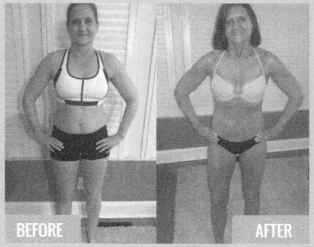

BEFORE   **AFTER**

CHANDLER B.

I'm also really proud of Chandler (55), who dropped nearly 14 pounds, 6 percent body fat, and 2 dress sizes in just three months:

"It took a couple weeks to kick in," she told me afterward, "but when it did, I saw progress every week, both in my body composition and the weight I was lifting."

CASSANDRA M.

Cassandra (38) also killed it, reducing her waist size by 5 inches and weight by 25 pounds in 12 weeks. Since a picture is worth a thousand words and all that . . .

"I am definitely more confident and feeling better about myself," she said afterward. "I am feeling just better overall. Definitely have more energy and determination."

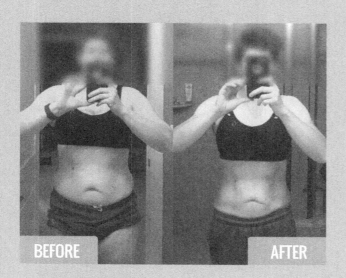

BEFORE   **AFTER**

Now, what about YOU?

Do you want to make this the year that you finally get super fit?

Are you ready to transform YOUR body and life?

If so, then you need to visit the URL below and schedule your free consultation call to see if my coaching service is right for you:

Go here now
→ www.muscleforlife.com/coaching

You have to hurry, though, because my coaches are always in high demand and availability is always limited.

This will NOT be a high-pressure sales call, by the way. It's a friendly chat where we get to learn where you're at, where you've been, and where you want to be, and then determine whether the program is right for you.

You should also know that this program comes with a very simple money-back guarantee:

You either love the experience and are thrilled with your results, or you get every penny you've paid back.

That's how much confidence I have in my team's ability to help you get great results.

So, take the first step in your journey to a new fitter, happier, and healthier you. Schedule your call now.

THE THINNER LEANER STRONGER EXERCISES

We are what we repeatedly do.
Greatness then is not an act, but a habit.

—ARISTOTLE

Out of the hundreds of resistance training exercises that you can do, a minority stand head and shoulders above the rest.

And out of those, a handful are the absolute breadwinners.

This is great news for us because it means we can disregard most of what we see people doing in magazines, YouTube videos, and the gym, and focus on getting really strong on a relatively short list of exercises instead.

In this chapter, I'm going to share those superior exercises with you, separated by major muscle group, as well as a refresher on proper form on the "Big Three" (the barbell squat, deadlift, and bench press).

THE BEST LEG EXERCISES YOU CAN DO

- *Barbell Squat*
- *Barbell Front Squat*
- *Hack Squat (Sled, Not Barbell)*
- *Single-Leg Split Squat (Barbell or Dumbbell)*
- *Leg Press*
- *Lunge (Dumbbell or Barbell, Walking or In-Place, Forward or Reverse)*
- *Romanian Deadlift*
- *Leg Curl (Lying or Seated)**
- *Standing Calf Raise*
- *Seated Calf Raise*
- *Leg Press Calf Raise*

THE BEST GLUTE EXERCISES YOU CAN DO

- *Barbell Squat*
- *Barbell Front Squat*
- *Barbell Deadlift*
- *Romanian Deadlift*
- *Lunge (Dumbbell or Barbell, Walking or In-Place, Forward or Reverse)*
- *Single-Leg Split Squat (Barbell or Dumbbell)*
- *Hip Thrust (Barbell or Dumbbell)*
- *Glute Blaster*
- *Step-Up (Barbell or Dumbbell)*
- *Weighted Back Hyperextension*

THE BEST CORE EXERCISES YOU CAN DO

- *Captain's Chair Leg Raise*
- *Hanging Leg Raise*
- *Lying Leg Raise*
- *Crunch*
- *Cable Crunch*
- *Weighted Sit-Up*
- *Plank*
- *Abdominal Rollout*

THE BEST BICEPS EXERCISES YOU CAN DO

- *Barbell Curl*
- *E-Z Bar Curl*
- *Alternating Dumbbell Curl*
- *Dumbbell Hammer Curl*
- *Chin-Up*

THE BEST TRICEPS EXERCISES YOU CAN DO

- *Close-Grip Bench Press*
- *Seated Triceps Press*
- *Dip*
- *Lying Triceps Extension ("Skullcrusher")*
- *Triceps Pushdown*

THE BEST SHOULDER EXERCISES YOU CAN DO

- *Overhead Press*
- *Military Press*
- *Seated Dumbbell Press*
- *Arnold Dumbbell Press*
- *Dumbbell Front Raise*
- *Dumbbell Side Lateral Raise*
- *Dumbbell Rear Lateral Raise (Bent-Over or Seated)*
- *Barbell Rear Delt Row*

THE BEST CHEST EXERCISES YOU CAN DO

- *Barbell Bench Press (Incline and Flat)*
- *Dumbbell Bench Press (Incline and Flat)*
- *Dip*
- *Cable Fly*

THE BEST BACK EXERCISES YOU CAN DO

- *Barbell Deadlift*
- *Barbell Row*
- *One-Arm Dumbbell Row*
- *Pull-Up*
- *Chin-Up*
- *T-Bar Row*
- *Lat Pulldown (Wide- and Close-Grip)*
- *Seated Cable Row (Wide- and Close-Grip)*

THE BARBELL SQUAT

There's a reason the barbell squat reigns supreme among weightlifting purists.

It requires over 200 muscles in the body to work together to generate a tremendous amount of force, as well as near-perfect form if you're going to ever put up impressive numbers.

And this is why the barbell squat is one of the single best exercises for developing every major muscle group in your body, from beak to butt.

THE SETUP

The best place to squat is in a power rack or squat rack with the safety bars or arms set to about six inches beneath your knees.

Position the bar on the rack so it cuts across the upper half of your chest. This might feel a bit low, but it's better to be on the low side than tippy-toeing the weight off the rack.

There are two ways to perform the barbell squat:
1. High-bar
2. Low-bar

A high-bar squat has the bar resting directly on the upper traps, whereas a low-bar position has the bar resting between the upper traps and rear deltoids.

Here's how they look:

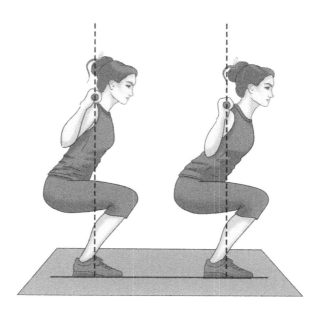

As you can see, your torso remains more upright in the high-bar squat.

Both methods are correct, but most people will find themselves stronger in the low-bar position because it allows you to better leverage your large leg muscles. That said, some people find the low-bar position very uncomfortable for their shoulders or wrists and naturally prefer the high-bar position.

If you're new to the barbell squat, I recommend you start with the low-bar position and only go high bar if it's too uncomfortable.

The barbell squat starts with approaching the weight and getting into position.

To do this, face the bar so you can walk it out backward. Don't ever walk the bar out forward, as trying to rerack it by walking backward is dangerous.

Get under the bar, get it into your preferred position, and place your feet about shoulder width apart, with the toes rotated out by about 20 to 25 degrees (your right foot should be at about 1 o'clock and your left at about 11 o'clock).

Next, place your thumbs on top of the bar and adjust your grip position. A narrow grip is preferable because it helps you maintain upper-back tightness, so get your hands as close together as you can, making sure your shoulder blades are pinched and the weight is solidly on your back muscles, not in your hands or resting on your spine.

Then, unrack the bar, take one or two steps back, and get back into the proper squatting position I've outlined (feet shoulder width apart, toes pointed out), and you're ready to descend.

THE DESCENT

Stand tall with your chest out and take a deep breath of air, pulling it into the bottom of your stomach (as opposed to your chest). Brace your abs as if you were about to get punched.

Pick a spot on the floor about six feet away and stare at it during the entire set. Don't look at the ceiling, as this makes it harder to reach the proper depth, can throw off proper hip movement and chest positioning, and can even cause a neck injury.

Begin the descent by simultaneously pushing your hips back and bending your knees. Don't consciously do one or the other first. You should feel backward motion in your hips and the sensation that you're sitting down between your heels.

Then, sit your butt straight down while keeping your chest up and back straight and tight. Your knees should point at your toes the whole way down (no bowing in!) and move forward for the first third or half of the movement, but no further than just in front of your toes.

Many people tend to want to slide their knees too far forward as they descend, which further loads the quads and puts the knees in a compromised position.

Descending too quickly increases the amount of force placed on your knees, so don't just drop your hips down as quickly as you can.[1] Make sure your descent is controlled.

The bottom of the squat is the point where your thighs are parallel to the ground or slightly lower. Your knees should still be pointing at your toes and over or slightly in front of them, and your back should be straight and at an angle that places the bar over the middle of your feet.

Here's how the bottom position looks:

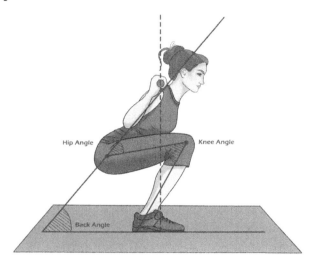

You're now ready to ascend.

THE ASCENT

The key to starting a good ascent is driving through your heels and the middle of your feet, and ensuring that your shoulders move upward at the same rate as your hips.

It also helps to imagine you're gripping the floor with your toes and feet, like an eagle clenching its claws.

As you continue to ascend, drive your hips forward by squeezing your glutes, and push the bar toward the ceiling until you're standing tall.

Begin exhaling once you've passed the hardest point of the ascent (the first couple of feet).

---

1. Myer GD, Kushner AM, Brent JL, et al. The back squat: A proposed assessment of functional deficits and technical factors that limit performance. *Strength Cond J.* 2014;36(6):4-27. doi:10.1519/SSC.0000000000000103.

Here's how the sequence looks:

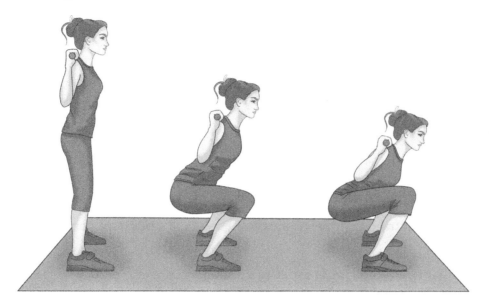

You're now ready for the next rep.

SIX TIPS FOR BETTER SQUATTING

1 **If you're having trouble keeping your knees in line with your toes, do the following mobility exercise every day.**

Without a bar or weight, squat down to the bottom position, and place your elbows against your knees and touch the palms of your hands together.

Use your elbows to press your knees out and into the proper position (in line with your toes), and hold this position for 20 to 30 seconds, followed by a minute or so of rest. Repeat this several times.

If you do this simple exercise every day, you should notice a marked improvement in your ability to maintain proper knee position when you squat in the gym.

2 **Don't squat on a Smith machine unless you have no other choice.**

The Smith machine forces you into an unnatural movement pattern that can be very uncomfortable, and research shows it's less effective than the free weight barbell squat.[2]

---

2. Schwanbeck S, Chilibeck PD, Binsted G. A Comparison of Free Weight Squat to Smith Machine Squat Using Electromyography. *J Strength Cond Res.* 2009;23(9):2588-2591. doi:10.1519/JSC.0b013e3181b1b181.

③ If you can't keep your lower-back in a neutral position as you descend because it begins to round, it's possible that your hamstrings are too tight or your that back isn't strong enough.

This is known as "butt wink," and in many people, it can be resolved through daily hamstring stretching (standing with one leg crossed over the other and then touching your toes, and reversing and repeating, works well).

As your hamstrings loosen, you'll find it much easier to keep your lower-back in a neutral position until you hit the very bottom of the squat, when your pelvis naturally rotates down a little.

Don't stretch before your squatting, though, because this can sap your strength.[3] Save it for after your lower-body workouts, when your muscles are nice and warm.

If you're confident hamstring tightness isn't the problem, it's possible you need to strengthen your back muscles.

In this case, you just need to be more mindful of making sure you don't add weight to the bar until you can maintain a neutral lower-back throughout each rep of each set.

Over time, your weaker back muscles will catch up to your stronger leg and hip muscles.

④ Don't squat with plates or blocks underneath your feet.

This doesn't make the exercise more effective and isn't a worthwhile variation to include in your workouts. That said, by elevating your heels while squatting, you can improve your form and range of motion.

Some people's hips are built in such a way that it makes it harder to safely and comfortably reach the bottom of the squat with good form. By slightly elevating your heels, you can change the mechanics of the squat enough to work around this limitation and perform the movement properly.

The best solution for this is to get a good pair of squat shoes, which have slightly elevated heels.

In fact, you should do this regardless of how comfortably you can squat, because the wrong shoes can make it significantly harder to progress.

Anything with a soft or unstable sole, like running shoes, shouldn't be used when squatting because it doesn't provide a solid, stable base through which you can transfer force into the floor.

Shoes with flat, solid soles and rigid, slightly elevated heels are much better because they allow for maximum force transfer. They also make it easier to maintain your balance as you descend, and they engage your hamstrings and glutes as you ascend.

---

3. Kay AD, Blazevich AJ. Effect of Acute Static Stretch on Maximal Muscle Performance. *Med Sci Sport Exerc.* 2012;44(1):154-164. doi:10.1249/ MSS.0b013e318225cb27.

5 Use the Valsalva maneuver to control your breathing.

The Valsalva maneuver is the process of forcefully breathing out against a closed windpipe. This traps air in your lungs and creates pressure inside your abdomen, known as intra-abdominal pressure, which stabilizes your torso against heavy loads.

Research shows that this increased intra-abdominal pressure allows you to lift more weight than you could with continuous breathing, and probably reduces the risk of injury as well.[4]

That's why the Valsalva maneuver is a useful technique for all exercises, not just the squat. Here's how to do it:

1. Take a deep breath of about 80 percent of your maximum lung capacity. Your belly should feel "full" but not so much that you have trouble keeping your mouth closed when the rep gets hard.

2. Press your tongue against the roof of your mouth, and without letting any air escape, try to breathe out. You should feel your abdomen, back, and jaw tighten.

3. Start your descent.

4. Once you're past the "sticking point" (the most difficult point) of the ascent, breathe out as you finish the rep.

5. Repeat for each rep in your set.

An important caveat: the Valsalva maneuver increases your blood pressure more than continuous breathing.

A number of studies show that this isn't inherently dangerous, and holding your breath is instinctive when lifting heavy weights, but if you're hypertensive or have a preexisting heart condition, you should talk with your doctor before using the Valsalva maneuver.[5]

Furthermore, if you use the technique and experience chest pain, dizziness, or other red flags, you should stop using it and talk with your doctor.

6 Use helpful cues as needed.

Cues are short reminders athletes use to draw their attention to particular aspects of their performance, typically whatever they struggle with the most. Here are some of my favorite cues for good squatting:

– Keep your chest up.
– Throw the bar off your back.

4. Blanchard TW, Smith C, Grenier SG. In a dynamic lifting task, the relationship between cross-sectional abdominal muscle thickness and the corresponding muscle activity is affected by the combined use of a weightlifting belt and the Valsalva maneuver. *J Electromyogr Kinesiol.* 2016;28:99-103. doi:10.1016/j.jelekin.2016.03.006.
5. Hackett DA, Chow C-M. The Valsalva Maneuver. J Strength Cond Res. 2013;27(8):2338-2345. doi:10.1519/JSC.0b013e31827de07d; Fleck SJ, Dean LS. Resistance-training experience and the pressor response during resistance exercise. *J Appl Physiol.* 1987;63(1):116-120. doi:10.1152/jappl.1987.63.1.116.

- Grab the floor (with your feet).
- Force your hips under the bar.
- Push the floor apart.
- Bend the bar over your back.

You don't have to memorize these cues or chant them as you squat, but if you're struggling with a particular portion of the movement, one of them may help you correct the issue.

THE BARBELL DEADLIFT

If I could do only one exercise for the rest of my life, it would be the barbell deadlift.

Mark Rippetoe said it best in an article he published on my website Muscle for Life (www.muscleforlife.com/how-to-look-strong-deadlift):

The deadlift works just about every muscle group you want to develop, from your upper-back muscles down to your calves, and it forces you to get strong the right way, with the bar in your hands balanced on your feet.

THE SETUP

The deadlift starts with the bar on the floor, not on the rack or safety arms or pins.

Walk up to the bar, position your feet so they're slightly narrower than shoulder width apart with your toes pointed slightly out, and move the bar to the point where your shoulders are in line with or even slightly behind it.

This will put the bar somewhere between against your shins and over the middle of your feet. For taller or skinnier people, it'll probably place the bar against their shins. For shorter or thicker people, it'll place it somewhere around the middle of the feet.

Proper bar position is important because it allows for maximum leverage as you pull it up and back. If the bar is too close to your body and your shoulders are too far in front of it, you'll have to move it forward on the way up to get it over your knees. If it's too far from your body, you'll feel like you're going to fall forward and won't be able to drive upward through your heels.

Next, stand up tall with your chest out and take a deep breath of air into your belly (as opposed to your chest), bracing your abs as if you were about to get punched in the stomach.

Then, move down toward the bar by pushing your hips back, just as you do in the squat. Arch your lower-back slightly and keep your shoulders down as you wedge yourself into what's essentially a "half-squat" position.

You should feel considerable tightness in your hamstrings and hips as you get into this position.

This is desirable because as soon as your hips rise, your shoulders will be able to follow, and the weight will immediately start coming off the floor.

Don't make the newbie mistake of bringing your hips too low with the intention of "squatting" the weight up. The lower your hips are in the starting position, the more they'll have to rise before you can lift the weight off the floor, which wastes movement and energy.

Next, place your hands on the bar with a double-overhand grip (both palms facing down) just outside your shins, and squeeze it as hard as you can. Keep your shoulders back and down and press your upper arms into your sides as if you were trying to crush oranges in your armpits.

Your arms should be completely straight and locked, with enough room on the sides for your thumbs to clear your thighs as you ascend.

Make sure your head is in a neutral position. Don't look up at the ceiling or down at the ground.

Here's how you should look:

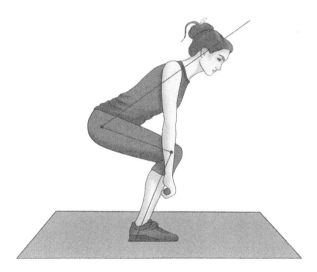

You're now ready to ascend.

THE ASCENT

Start the pull by forcefully driving your body upward and slightly back, onto your heels. Push through your heels, and keep your elbows locked in place and lower-back slightly arched (no rounding!).

Ensure that your hips and shoulders rise simultaneously. Don't shoot your hips up and then use your back like a lever to raise your shoulders. If your hips are moving up, your shoulders should be as well.

The bar should move up your shins, and once it rolls over your knees, push your hips into the bar. As it begins to move up your thighs, you'll feel your hamstrings and hips working hard as you continue to stand.

The entire way up, keep your head in its neutral position in line with your spine, your lower-back slightly arched, and your core tight. Also, try to keep the bar on as vertically straight of a path as possible because any deviations are just going to slow you down and make it harder to maintain good form. The bar shouldn't move noticeably toward or away from you.

At the top, your chest should be up and your shoulders down. Don't lean back, hyperextend your lower-back, or shrug the weight up.

Here's how this movement looks:

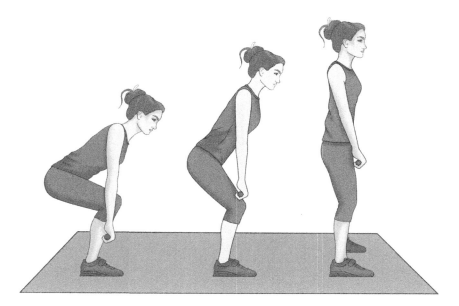

You're now ready to descend

THE DESCENT

The next half of the deadlift is lowering the weight back down to the floor in a controlled manner. This is basically a mirror image of what you did to stand up.

Begin by pushing your hips back, not bending at the knees, letting the bar slide straight down your thighs. Continue pushing your hips back, lowering the bar in a straight line until it has cleared your knees, and then drop it to the floor.

Your lower-back should remain locked in its neutral position the entire time, and your core should remain tight. Don't try to lower the bar slowly or quietly. The entire descent should take one to two seconds or less.

THE YEAR ONE CHALLENGE FOR WOMEN **45**

You're now ready for the next rep.

Many people don't stop to reset in between reps and instead use the tap-and-go transition, which has you maintain tension as you tap the weights to the floor and immediately begin the next rep.

This is fine if you're warming up, but I prefer the stop-and-go method for my hard sets. This method has you fully release the weight to the ground and reset your bottom position—including your breath—before starting the next rep. This is harder than tap-and-go, but that's good, and it's safer as well.

THE ROMANIAN DEADLIFT

The main differences between the Romanian and conventional deadlift are:

1. You can start with the bar in a power rack instead of on the floor (but don't have to).
2. Your legs remain fairly straight, bending only slightly at the knees to lower the bar.
3. You lower the bar to just below your knees or when your lower-back starts to round, and no further.

Let's go through technique.

THE SETUP

There are two ways to set up for the Romanian deadlift:

1. From the rack
2. From the floor

If you start from the rack, you'll want the bar to be just below where you'll hold it at the top of the movement, or about midthigh.

If you start from the floor, then all you have to do is set up the same way you would for the conventional deadlift.

Most people prefer starting from the rack because it makes it easier to load the bar and doesn't force you to waste energy pulling it off the floor at the beginning of each set.

To set up, walk up to the bar so that it's over the middle of your feet, position your feet about shoulder width apart with your toes pointed slightly out, and grip the bar with a double-overhand grip.

Next, take a deep breath, raise your chest, and press your upper arms into your sides as if you were trying to crush oranges in your armpits.

Lift the bar off the rack (or floor), take a baby step back if you're coming from the rack, and bend your knees slightly. Fix your gaze on a spot about 10 feet in front of you.

You're now ready to descend.

THE DESCENT

To descend, allow your hips to move backward as you lower the bar down the front of your legs.

As the bar drops down in a straight line, keep your knees at more or less the same angle as when you started. Once you start to feel a stretch in your hamstrings, you can allow slightly more bend in your knees.

At this point, the bar should be at knee height or just below.

Don't try to lower the bar to the ground. Doing so forces you to bend your knees even more, which reduces tension on the hamstrings and defeats the purpose of the exercise.

Once you can't go any lower without rounding your lower-back or further bending your knees, you're ready to ascend.

THE ASCENT

Keeping your back and core tight, chest up, and knees slightly bent, drive your hips forward while pulling the bar straight up.

Here's how this movement looks:

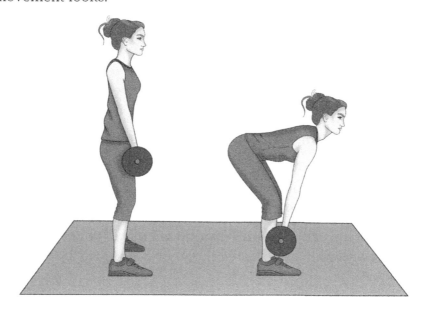

Once you're standing tall, you're ready for the next rep.

SIX TIPS FOR BETTER DEADLIFTING

1 Squeeze the bar as hard as you can.

Try to crush it with your hands. If your knuckles aren't white, you're not squeezing hard enough.

2 Boost your grip.

Grip weakness not only makes the bar harder to hold onto, it shuts down the entire exercise. Once the bar starts rolling out of your hands, you'll grind to a halt.

Your grip will get stronger as you train, but chances are it's going to fall behind the rest of your body in your deadlift and become a limiting factor.

A common workaround is the "mixed grip," which involves alternating one of your hands so it's palm-up. This works well but also has downsides:

1. It makes you tend to rotate your torso toward your palm-down hand, creating a load imbalance between the left and right sides of your body.

2. It places more strain on the biceps of your palm-up arm.[6]

I don't know of any scientific data on how this affects the safety of the exercise, but I'll say this: while biceps tears are rare, when they do happen, it's often from the palm-up biceps during a heavy mixed-grip deadlift.

You can take a simple precaution to make the mixed grip safer—alternate your palm-up hand in individual workouts or between them—but I'd rather you just use a double-overhand grip with straps instead.

Many people shy away from straps because they look at them as a form of "cheating," but this is silly. When used properly, straps allow you to safely pull more weight without any of the downsides of the mixed grip (and its excruciating cousin, the hook grip, which we won't even discuss because of what it does to your thumbs).

To use straps, pick up some simple lasso straps, pull without them until your grip starts to give out (your second or third hard set, for instance), and then use them to finish up. Straps can help with barbell and dumbbell rows, too.

You can also include grip exercises in your routine at any point if you're so inclined. My favorite is the plain ol' barbell hold, which is exactly what it sounds like: holding onto a heavy barbell.

Here's how to do it:

1. Using a squat rack, place the bar at your knees and load it with a weight you can hold for no more than 15 to 20 seconds.

2. Do three sets of 15-to-20-second holds, resting for three minutes between each set.

---

6. Beggs LA. Comparison of muscle activation and kinematics during the deadlift using a double-pronated and overhand/underhand grip. *University of Kentucky Master's Theses.* 2011.

Do this once or twice per week at the end of workouts, separated by two to three days. You should see marked improvements within your first month or so.

Last but not least, you can also use weightlifting chalk for an easy boost in your grip strength. Chalk helps by absorbing sweat and increasing the friction between your palms and the bar, and you can go with the liquid variety if you don't want to make a mess or your gym doesn't allow it.

3 Use the right shoes.

As with squatting, deadlifting in shoes that have foam or air cushions or gel fillings compromises your stability, power production, and form.

Plus, most athletic shoes aren't made for deadlifting and fall apart after just a few months of regular use. Deadlift in your squat shoes instead, in shoes with flat, hard soles, or in socks.

4 Explode up from the floor.

Don't start the pull slowly. This makes it easier to get stuck. Instead, shoot your body up as quickly as you can by applying maximum force to the ground through your heels.

5 Wear shin guards, knee-length socks, or knee sleeves.

For most people, proper deadlifting form requires pulling the bar up their shins, which starts to tear them up as weights get heavy. ("Are her shins bleeding?")

You can wear pants or tights, but they're going to get shredded over time.

This is why I recommend protecting your shins while you deadlift with lightweight shin guards, knee-length socks, or a pair of knee sleeves that you wear below your knees.

6 Use the Valsalva maneuver to control your breathing.

As you learned, this helps stabilize your torso against heavy loads, which helps you safely move more weight. That's why it's useful for all compound exercises.

In the case of the deadlift, you can breathe out after the bar clears the midthighs.

THE BARBELL BENCH PRESS

The barbell bench press is one of the best all-around upper-body exercises you can do, training the pectorals, lats, shoulders, triceps, and even the legs to a slight degree.

THE SETUP

First, lie down on the bench and adjust yourself so your eyes are under the bar.

Then, raise your chest up and tuck your shoulder blades down and squeeze them together. Think of pulling your shoulder blades into your back pockets. This should produce tightness in your upper-back.

Next, grab the bar with your hands slightly wider than shoulder width apart, about 14 to 20 inches, depending on your build. If you go too narrow, you'll shift the emphasis to the triceps instead of the pecs, and if you go too wide, you'll reduce the range of motion and effectiveness of the exercise and increase the risk of irritating your shoulders.

Hold the bar low in your hands, closer to your wrists than your fingers, and squeeze it as hard as you can. Your wrists should be bent just enough to allow the bar to settle into the base of your palm, but not folded back toward your head.

Here's how this looks:

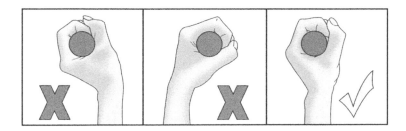

A good way to check your grip width is to have a friend get behind you and check the position of your forearms at the bottom of the movement. You want your forearms to be as close to straight up-and-down vertical as possible, like this:

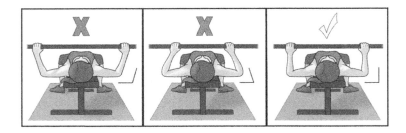

As you can see, the position on the far left is too wide, the middle is too narrow, and the far right is correct.

Don't use a "thumbless" or "suicide" grip (as it's aptly called), where your thumbs are next to your index fingers instead of wrapped around the bar.

When you're going heavy, this grip can make it surprisingly easy for the bar to slip out of your hands and crash down on your chest, or worse, your neck.

Next, slightly arch your lower-back and plant your feet on the ground, directly under your knees, about shoulder width apart.

You don't want your back flat on the bench and you don't want it so arched that your butt is floating above it. Instead, you want to maintain the natural arch that occurs when you push your chest out.

The upper part of your leg should be parallel to the floor, and the lower part should be perpendicular (forming a 90-degree angle). This allows you to push through your heels as you ascend, creating a "leg drive" that'll boost your strength.

Then, unrack the bar by locking your elbows out and moving it off the hooks horizontally until it's directly over your shoulders. Don't try to bring the weight directly from the hooks to your chest, and don't drop your chest and loosen your shoulder blades when unracking.

Finally, with the bar in place, take a deep breath, push your knees apart, and squeeze the bar.

You're now ready to descend.

THE DESCENT

The first thing you should know about the descent is how to tuck your elbows properly.

Many people make the mistake of flaring them out (away from the body), which can cause a shoulder injury. A less common mistake is tucking your elbows too close to your torso, which robs you of stability and strength and can aggravate your elbows.

Instead, you want your elbows to remain at a 30-to-60-degree angle relative to your torso throughout the entire movement. This protects your shoulders from injury and provides a stable, strong position to press from.

Here's a helpful visual:

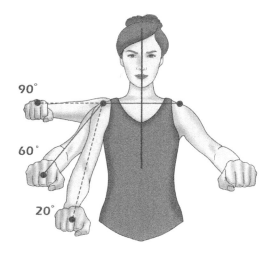

As you can see, in the bottommost position, the arms are at about a 20-degree angle relative to the torso, which is too close. The middle position is the ideal one—about 45 degrees—and the topmost is the undesirable 90 degrees.

Keeping your elbows tucked and in place, lower the bar to the lower part of your chest, over your nipples. The bar should move in a straight line down, not toward your face or belly button.

Once the bar has touched your chest (touched, not bounced off), you're ready to ascend.

THE ASCENT

Although it's called the bench press, it's better to think of it as pushing rather than pressing.

That is, picture that you're pushing your torso away from the bar and into the bench instead of pressing the bar away from your body. This will help you maintain proper form and maximize power.

Keeping your shoulder blades down and pinched, your elbows tucked, your lower-back slightly arched, your butt on the bench, and your feet on the floor, push against the bar to get it off your chest.

You can also utilize the "leg drive" I mentioned earlier by pressing your heels into the floor and spreading your knees as you begin to push the bar. This transfers force up through the hips and back, which helps with form and increases the amount of power you can generate.

The bar should move up in a slightly diagonal path, shifting toward and ending where you began—with it directly over your shoulders, where it's most naturally balanced.
Lock your elbows out at the top of the movement. Don't keep them slightly bent.

You're now ready for the next rep.

Once you've completed your final rep in a set, you're ready to rack the bar. Don't try to press the bar directly into the hooks because if you miss, it's coming down on your face.

Instead, finish your final rep with the bar directly over your shoulders and your elbows locked, and then move the bar horizontally into the uprights.

THE CLOSE-GRIP BENCH PRESS

At bottom, the close-grip bench press is just a regular bench press but with a narrower grip. Other than the grip modification, you should perform the close-grip bench press in exactly the same way as the regular bench press.

For your grip, your hands should be slightly (a few inches) inside your shoulders. Some people place their hands just a few inches apart to try to maximize the triceps' involvement, but this puts the shoulders and wrists in a potentially dangerous position.

If your shoulders or wrists feel uncomfortable at the bottom of the movement (when the bar is touching your chest), simply widen your grip by about the width of a finger on each side and try again. Repeat until it's comfortable.

SIX TIPS FOR BETTER BENCH PRESSING

1 **Don't watch the bar as it moves.**

Watching the bar will likely vary its angles of descent and ascent, which wastes energy. Instead, pick a spot on the ceiling to look at during the exercise and see the bar going down and up in relation to it. The goal is to bring the bar up to the same spot in each rep.

2 **Try to pull the bar down and apart.**

This is an old-school powerlifting tip that has been proven to work in scientific research. The idea is simple:

1. Don't start the descent by letting the bar drop toward your body.

Instead, imagine you're pulling the bar down toward your chest in a controlled manner. This will help you maintain the proper body position for generating maximum vertical force.[7]

2. As you descend, try to bend the bar in half or "pull it apart." This requires keeping your shoulder blades in their proper position (pulled in toward each other).

Applying lateral force in this way also helps you generate more vertical force when you ascend, which is one of the reasons you can move more weight on the barbell bench press than dumbbell press.[8] You can't generate lateral force with dumbbells because they simply move away from each other.

3 **Keep your butt on the bench at all times.**

If your butt is lifting off the bench, the weight is probably too heavy.

The three points of contact you should always maintain for optimal bench pressing are the upper-back (down on the bench), the butt (ditto), and the feet (always planted on the floor squarely beneath your knees).

4 **Don't smash the back of your head into the bench.**

This can strain your neck. Your neck will naturally tighten while doing the exercise, but don't forcefully push it down.

5 **When you're lowering the weight, think about the ascent.**

Visualize the explosive second half of the exercise the entire time, and you'll find it easier to control the descent, prevent bouncing, and even prepare your muscles for the stress of raising the bar.

(This technique works well for all exercises, by the way.)

---

7. Duffey MJ, Challis JH. Vertical and Lateral Forces Applied to the Bar during the Bench Press in Novice Lifters. *Lifters. J Strength Cond Res.* 2011;25(9):2442-2447. doi:10.1519/JSC.0b013e3182281939; Madsen N, McLaughlin T. Kinematic factors influencing performance and injury risk in the bench press exercise. *Med Sci Sports Exerc.* 1984;16(4):376-381.

8. Duffey MJ, Challis JH. Vertical and Lateral Forces Applied to the Bar during the Bench Press in Novice *Lifters. J Strength Cond Res.* 2011;25(9):2442-2447. doi:10.1519/JSC.0b013e3182281939.

THE YEAR ONE CHALLENGE FOR WOMEN **53**

6 **Use the Valsalva maneuver to control your breathing.**

As I mentioned previously, I recommend you use the Valsalva maneuver during all your compound exercises, and that includes the bench press.

In this case, you can breathe out after the bar is about four to six inches above your chest.

THE THINNER LEANER STRONGER CHEAT SHEET

I love to see a young girl go out and grab the world by the lapels.
Life's a bitch. You've got to go out and kick ass.

—MAYA ANGELOU

Thinner Leaner Stronger isn't complex as far as weightlifting programs go, but it does have a number of moving parts that make it work.

In this chapter you'll find concise information on the program's key points, to which you can refer back at any time until everything sinks in and becomes second nature.

WARMING UP

To ensure that each of the major muscle groups you're going to train in a workout is warmed up and primed for optimum performance, you're going to do several warm-up sets with the first exercises for each of those muscle groups.

Here's an easy and effective routine that will warm you up without doing so much that your performance on your hard sets is compromised:

1. Do 10 reps with about 50 percent of your hard set weight, and rest for a minute.

2. Do 10 reps with the same weight at a slightly faster pace, and rest for a minute.

3. Do 4 reps with about 70 percent of your hard set weight, and rest for a minute.

And that's it. You're now ready to do your hard sets.

REP RANGE

Thinner Leaner Stronger is going to have you work in the rep range of 8 to 10 reps, meaning that most hard sets for all exercises are going to entail doing at least 8 reps but not more than 10. For most women, this means working with weights that are around 70 to 75 percent of their one-rep max.

DOUBLE PROGRESSION

When you get 10 reps for one hard set, you immediately move up in weight by adding 5 pounds to the bar or moving up to dumbbells that are 5 pounds heavier (per dumbbell).

Remember the example of how this works in *Thinner Leaner Stronger*?

Let's say you're squatting in the 8-to-10-rep range, and on your first (or second) hard set of your workout, you get 10 reps with 100 pounds. You then immediately move up in weight by adding 5 pounds to the bar or moving up to dumbbells that are 5 pounds heavier (per dumbbell).

Great! The progression has succeeded, and you now work with 105 pounds in your current and future workouts until you can squat it for one hard set of 10 reps. Then, you'd move up in weight again, and so on.

What if you only get 5 or 6 reps with the new, heavier weight before your form starts breaking down? What if the progression doesn't succeed?

In this case, you should drop the weight back to the original, lighter load (100 pounds in our example) and work there until you can squat it for two hard sets of 10 reps (in the same workout).

Then, you should immediately move up to the heavier weight again on your next hard set (even if that's in your next workout) and try again.

If you do that and still can't get at least 7 reps, go back to the lighter weight and work with it until you can do three hard sets of 10 reps (in the same workout). At this point, your progression should succeed.

Also, if you get 10 reps in your first set after moving up in weight, then you get to move up again!

And what should you do if you get 10 reps on your third and final hard set for an exercise in your workout? You should increase the weight on your first hard set of your next performance of that exercise.

Finally, if your gym doesn't have 2.5-pound plates, then you can add 10 pounds to the bar when you move up in weight.

SET INTENSITY

You want to end each of your hard sets one or two reps shy of technical failure, which again, is the point where you can't do another rep with proper form.

REP TEMPO

Follow the traditional "1–1–1" rep tempo for all weightlifting exercises.

This means the first part of each rep (either the eccentric, or lengthening phase, or in some cases, the concentric, or contraction phase) should take about one second, followed by a one-second (or shorter) pause, followed by the final part of the rep, which should also take about one second.

For example, if we apply this to the squat, it would mean sitting to the proper depth in about one second, pausing for a moment, and standing up quickly.

RESTING IN BETWEEN SETS

You want to rest around three minutes in between each hard set.

You can rest slightly less (two minutes) in between hard sets for smaller muscle groups like the biceps, triceps, and shoulders, and slightly more (four minutes) in between hard sets for your larger muscle groups like your back and legs if your heart rate hasn't settled down, or if you simply feel you need a little more time before you can give maximum effort on your next hard set.

EXERCISE SEQUENCE

Do the exercises in a workout one at a time and complete all the hard sets for one exercise before moving on to another, like this:

If you can't do an exercise in a workout for whatever reason, simply choose an alternative "approved" exercise from the previous chapter to take its place, or do three more sets of an exercise already in your workout.

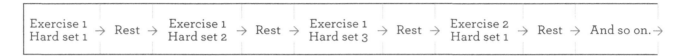

CORE TRAINING

CAPTAIN'S CHAIR LEG RAISE

This exercise is normally unweighted, but you can add weight by holding a dumbbell in between your feet as you raise and lower them.

Here's how I like to approach this exercise:

1. Start unweighted.

2. Take all hard sets to technical failure.

3. Once you can do at least 30 reps before failing, turn it into a weighted exercise by snatching a dumbbell in between your feet. Start with 10 pounds.

4. Once you do 30 reps with 10 pounds, go up by 5 pounds.

5. Continue progressing in this way.

If you reach the point where adding more weight becomes awkward, then it's time to switch to a different exercise, like the hanging leg raise.

HANGING LEG RAISE

This exercise is a harder variation of the captain's chair leg raise, and I recommend going about it in the same way.

LYING LEG RAISE
—

This exercise is similar to the previous two but doesn't require any equipment.

Once you can do at least 50 reps in a single hard set before reaching technical failure, start doing weighted captain's chair or hanging leg raises instead.

CRUNCH
—

This is a staple ab exercise that should be done unweighted and to technical failure in each hard set.

Once you can do at least 50 reps in a single hard set before reaching technical failure, start doing weighted sit-ups or cable crunches instead.

CABLE CRUNCH
—

I recommend the 8-to-10-rep range for all hard sets of cable crunches and increasing the weight in 5- or 10-pound increments.

Furthermore, you should treat this exercise exactly the same as any other resistance training exercise—your goal is to get stronger over time, you rest a couple of minutes in between sets, you use a 1-1-1 rep tempo, and so on.

WEIGHTED SIT-UP
—

This weighted exercise allows you to effectively train your abdominal muscles with free weights.

As previously noted, I recommend you work up to 50 unweighted crunches before moving on to weighted sit-ups.

As with the cable crunch, work in the 8-to-10-rep range on this exercise and increase the weight in 5- or 10-pound increments.

As with the cable crunch, you should treat this exercise exactly the same as any other resistance training exercise—your goal is to get stronger over time, you rest a couple of minutes in between sets, you use a 1-1-1 rep tempo, and so on.

Also, you may see some people hold the weight behind their necks while doing this exercise. This can work with light weights but becomes uncomfortable and even dangerous with heavier weights, so keep the weight on your chest instead.

PLANK

—

This is another effective unweighted exercise for training the back and core muscles.

Start by holding a hard set for as long as you can before reaching technical failure. Then, try to increase the amount of time you can hold the plank position by five seconds per workout.

Once you can do at least one two-minute hard set of the basic plank, you can increase the difficulty by making two small adjustments:[1]

Instead of positioning your elbows directly under your shoulders, extend them three to six inches in front of your shoulders.

Instead of relaxing your glutes, flex them as if you were doing a hip thrust.

Once you can do one two-minute hard set of the modified plank, start doing a more difficult exercise instead, like the cable crunch, abdominal rollout, or weighted sit-up.

ABDOMINAL ROLLOUT

—

The abdominal rollout is a classic unweighted ab exercise that deserves a place in your repertoire.

Start this exercise on your knees, and once you can do at least 30 reps before reaching technical failure, increase the difficulty by remaining on your feet, like a plank.

Once you can do at least 30 reps on your feet before reaching technical failure, start doing weighted sit-ups or cable crunches instead.

AVOIDING INJURY

IF IT HURTS, DON'T DO IT

—

I'm not talking about muscle soreness or the burning sensation that occurs as you approach technical failure, but pain. If a rep hurts enough to make you wince, that means you need to stop. Pain is a warning that something is wrong, and if you don't listen to it, you're asking for trouble. So, when you hit pain, stop, rest for a couple of minutes, and try the exercise again.

If it still hurts, do something else and come back to it next workout and see how it goes. If it's still a problem, substitute it with a different exercise. Don't think that you "have" to do any specific exercise in any workout, even if it hurts.

---

1. Schoenfeld BJ, Contreras B, Tiryaki-Sonmez G, Willardson JM, Fontana F. An electromyographic comparison of a modified version of the plank with a long lever and posterior tilt versus the traditional plank exercise. *Sport Biomech*. 2014;13(3):296-306. doi:10.1080/14763141.2014.942355.

If you aren't sure if what you're feeling qualifies as pain or the normal discomfort of training, ask yourself these two questions:

1 **Is the pain on both sides of my body or just one?**

When you perform exercises correctly, both sides of your body are fairly equally subjected to stress.

Thus, if one side starts to hurt more than the other, it's more likely a sign of trouble rather than merely muscle burn or fatigue.

2 **Is the pain concentrated around a joint or other specific spot?**

These are the types of pains that you're most likely to encounter because muscle strains and tears are uncommon.

Muscle and joint aches and stiffness generally go away if you warm up properly, but genuine pains won't (in fact, they'll often get worse).

Therefore, when localized pain strikes and lingers, back off and rest the affected area(s) until the pain is completely gone.

PROGRESS GRADUALLY
—

One of the easiest ways to get hurt in weightlifting is getting greedy.

Maybe you're feeling particularly strong one day, or you want to impress or one-up someone in the gym or just progress faster, so you load the bar with a weight that makes your spidey senses tingle.

This is almost always a bad idea. It increases the likelihood that your form will break down, it can place more stress on your joints and ligaments than they can safely handle, and it can make fully recovering from your training harder.

A much smarter, and ultimately more effective, approach to progression is one that's slow and steady.

If you're new to weightlifting and you can add five pounds to your big lifts every week or two for the first several months, you're doing great.

If you're an experienced weightlifter on a lean bulk, gaining just one rep per week on these exercises (and thus adding weight every few weeks) is good progress.

BE A STICKLER FOR GOOD FORM
—

Remember the goal in weightlifting isn't to haphazardly lift as much weight as possible, but to carefully control heavy loads through a full ranges of motion.
This not only protects you from injury but also makes every rep, exercise, and workout more conducive to muscle and strength gain.

This is especially important with compound exercises like the squat, deadlift, and bench press because while they're not inherently dangerous, they involve the heaviest weights and most technical skill.

There's a big difference between cheating on the last rep or two of isolation exercises like the dumbbell curl and lateral raise versus a barbell pull or press.

So, don't sacrifice form for the sake of progression. Instead, learn proper form for every exercise you do and stick to it.

TRACKING YOUR PROGRESS

To track changes in your body composition, you should do the following:

1. Weigh yourself daily and calculate weekly averages.
2. Take weekly body measurements.
3. Take weekly progress pictures.

The procedure here is easy:

1. Weigh yourself first thing in the morning, naked and after the bathroom and before eating or drinking anything.

2. Then, every seven days, add up your last seven weigh-ins and divide by seven to get your average daily weight for the last week.

3. Record your averages somewhere easily accessible, like an Excel or Google Sheet or the notepad app in your phone.

   If you want to take your weight-tracking game a step further, you can graph the numbers in Excel or Google Sheets.

As you're well aware, your weight can shoot up a few pounds during your period, so I recommend you watch the averages of the weeks before and after your period weeks to track your progress.

Record at least one body measurement every week in addition to your weight: your waist circumference.

To take this measurement, wrap a tape measure around your bare stomach, right at your navel. Make sure the tape measure is parallel to the floor (not slanted) and snug to your body, but not so tight that it compresses the skin. Exhale while taking the measurement, and don't flex or suck your stomach in.

Make sure you measure in the same spot every time so your readings stay consistent.

Hip circumference is another measurement some women like to take because it too is another reliable marker of fat loss or gain.

If you want to take it, do so when you measure your waist (once per week).

To take this measurement, wrap a tape measure around the widest point between the top of your hip bone and the bottom of your butt. This spot can vary from person to person depending on body composition, but it's generally right above your "naughty bits."

Make sure you measure in the same spot every time so your readings stay consistent.

And if you're the type of person who loves tracking data and quantifying things, here are two more measurements you can take:

→ Your upper-leg circumference

   To take this measurement, wrap a tape measure around the widest part of one of your leg's thigh and hamstrings. Then do the same for your other leg.

   Take these measurements every week with your other weekly measurements, and make sure you measure in the same spots every time.

→ Your flexed arms

   To take this measurement, flex one of your arms and wrap a tape measure around the largest part (the peak of your biceps and middle of your triceps). Then do the same for your other arm.

Take these measurements every week with your other weekly measurements, and make sure you measure in the same spots every time.

Take progress pictures every week when you take your weekly measurements.

Here's how to do it right:

→ Take pictures from the front, side, and back.

→ Show as much skin as you feel comfortable with. The more the better because it gives you the best idea of how your body is changing.

→ Use the same camera, lighting, and background for each picture. If you aren't able to do this, make sure the pictures are clear.

→ Take the pictures at the same time every day, preferably in the morning, after using the bathroom and before breakfast.

→ Take both flexed and unflexed pictures, as this lets you see how your muscles are developing.

I also recommend saving all your progress photos in an individual album on your phone or computer so as time goes on, you can easily scroll through them.

THE THINNER LEANER STRONGER MEAL PLANS

A woman is the full circle. Within her is the power to create, nurture and transform.

—DIANE MARIECHILD

Thinner Leaner Stronger isn't complex as far As you learned in *Thinner Leaner Stronger*, meal planning is much like putting together a jigsaw puzzle.

You can dump the pieces into a heap and try to muddle your way through it, or you can shortcut the process by being more systematic—start with the edges, sort the tabs and blanks, separate into color groups, and so forth.

If you want to brush up on meal planning, you can refer back to chapters 17 and 19 of *Thinner Leaner Stronger*, but here's the procedure in a nutshell:

1. Calculate your daily calorie target based on your goals.

2. Calculate your daily macronutrient targets based on your goals.

3. Load up the meal planning template in the free bonus material that comes with *Thinner Leaner Stronger* (www.thinnerleanerstronger.com/bonus), or you can use Excel or Google Sheets, or paper or notebook and a pen.

4. Create a list of your preferred foods and recipes.

5. Familiarize yourself with the nutritional facts of your food choices using CalorieKing, SELF Nutrition Data, or the USDA Food Composition databases.

6. Remove any foods or recipes that are too high-calorie or macronutritionally imbalanced to fit your needs.

7. Set up your pre- and post-workout meals first.

8. Add your primary sources of protein to the rest of your meals.

9. Add your fruits and vegetables.

10. Add any additional carbs and caloric beverages that aren't dessert or junk.

11. Tweak your protein intake as needed.

12. Add additional fat as needed.

13. Add treats if desired.

Remember that you want to be within 50 calories of your target intake when cutting and within 100 calories when lean bulking.

On the following pages you'll find several examples of effective and well-made meal plans for cutting, lean bulking, and maintaining, or you can refer to the examples found in the free bonus material that comes with *Thinner Leaner Stronger*.

CUTTING MEAL PLAN FOR A 160-POUND WOMAN

MEAL	FOOD	AMOUNT	CALORIES	PROTEIN	CARBS	FAT
PREWORKOUT MEAL	Plain nonfat Greek yogurt	340 grams	201	35	12	1
	Banana	136 grams	121	1	31	0
	TOTAL		322	36	43	1
WEIGHTLIFTING						
POSTWORKOUT SHAKE	Plain nonfat Greek yogurt	240 grams	142	24	9	1
	Unsweetened almond milk	240 grams	36	1	3	2
	Blueberry	140 grams	80	1	20	0
	Banana	136 grams	121	1	31	0
	TOTAL		379	27	63	3
LUNCH	Skinless boneless chicken breast	200 grams	240	45	0	5
	Fat-free refried bean	130 grams	120	7	22	0
	Reduced fat cheddar cheese	28 grams	49	7	1	2
	Onion	60 grams	60	19	0	5
	Tomato	120 grams	22	1	5	0
	Salsa	36 grams	10	1	2	0
	Olive oil	10 grams	88	0	0	10
	TOTAL		589	80	30	22
DINNER	Pork chop, trimmed of visible fat	200 grams	254	45	0	7
	Butternut squash	200 grams	90	2	23	0
	Broccoli	100 grams	34	3	7	0
	Cauliflower	100 grams	25	2	5	0
	Butter	10 grams	72	0	0	8
	TOTAL		475	52	35	15
	DAILY TOTAL		1,765	195	171	41
	DAILY TARGET		1,760	176	176	39

LEAN BULKING MEAL PLAN FOR A 100-POUND WOMAN

MEAL	FOOD	AMOUNT	CALORIES	PROTEIN	CARBS	FAT
PREWORKOUT MEAL	Egg white	100 grams	52	11	1	0
	Cooked bacon	13 grams	60	6	0	4
	Whole grain bread	28 grams	80	4	14	0
	Jam	20 grams	56	0	14	0
	Butter	5 grams	34	0	0	4
TOTAL			282	21	29	8
WEIGHTLIFTING						
POSTWORKOUT SHAKE	Plain nonfat Greek yogurt	170 grams	100	17	6	0
	Unsweetened rice milk	240 grams	113	1	22	2
	Banana	136 grams	121	2	31	1
	Blueberry	148 grams	84	1	22	1
TOTAL			418	21	81	4
LUNCH	Whole wheat pita bread	64 grams	168	6	36	1
	Reduced fat provolone cheese	14 grams	38	3	0	2
	Roasted turkey breast	100 grams	147	30	2	0
	Reduced fat mayonnaise	15 grams	50	0	1	5
	Mustard	10 grams	6	0	1	0
TOTAL			409	39	40	8
SNACK	Apple	182 grams	95	0	25	0
TOTAL			95	0	25	0
DINNER	Sirloin, trimmed of visible fat	100 grams	126	22	0	4
	Brown rice	80 grams	290	6	61	2
	75% dark chocolate	14 grams	85	1	7	6
TOTAL			429	29	68	12
DAILY TOTAL			1,705	110	243	32
DAILY TARGET			1,700	106	234	38

MAINTENANCE MEAL PLAN FOR A 130-POUND WOMAN

MEAL	FOOD	AMOUNT	CALORIES	PROTEIN	CARBS	FAT
PREWORKOUT MEAL	Whole egg	100 grams	143	13	1	10
	Egg white	130 grams	68	14	1	0
	Oat	40 grams	152	5	27	3
	Unsweetened almond milk	240 grams	36	1	3	2
	Strawberry	140 grams	45	1	11	0
TOTAL			444	34	43	15
WEIGHTLIFTING						
POSTWORKOUT SHAKE	Plain nonfat Greek yogurt	340 grams	201	35	12	1
	Banana	136 grams	121	2	31	1
	White bread	28 grams	74	3	14	1
	Avocado	60 grams	96	1	5	9
TOTAL			492	40	62	12
LUNCH	Chunky Chicken Quesadillas from *The Shredded Chef*	1 serving	315	30	28	9
TOTAL			315	30	28	9
SNACK	Grape	120 grams	83	1	22	0
TOTAL			83	1	22	0
DINNER	Farmed Atlantic salmon	112 grams	233	23	0	15
	Brown rice	70 grams	253	5	53	2
	Broccoli	300 grams	102	9	20	1
TOTAL			588	37	73	18
DAILY TOTAL			1,922	141	228	54
DAILY TARGET			1,950	146	219	54

THE THINNER LEANER STRONGER QUICKSTART GUIDE

Any airplane is off track much of the time
but just keeps coming back to the flight plan.

—STEPHEN R. COVEY

To make things as smooth as possible for you, I'm going to give you a comprehensive checklist that'll take you by the hand and get you up to speed fast.

This quickstart guide is broken down into eight major steps:

1. Buy your supplies.

2. Join or set up a gym.

3. Take your first measurements and pictures.

4. Create your first meal plan.

5. Create your workout schedule.

6. Prepare for your first week.

7. Do your first week.
8. Get ready for your next week (and beyond!).

Each of these steps has several substeps, including optional ones, which aren't necessary for following the program but are recommended for reasons you've learned about in this book.

Once you've done those eight things, you'll officially be on your way, so let's get to it!

1. BUY YOUR SUPPLIES

You don't need much in the way of gear and gadgets to follow Thinner Leaner Stronger, but you do need a few items, and you should consider picking up a few others as well.

You can find links to my specific product recommendations in the free bonus material that comes with this book (www.thinnerleanerstronger.com/bonus).

→ Buy a digital food scale and learn to use its basic functions, like switching between units and taring, because you need to be precise with your food intake.

→ OPTIONAL: Buy plastic containers to store your meals.

→ Any kind will do, but they should be BPA-free and microwave safe and have see-through lids and compartments. You can also get small containers for snacks, glass ones instead of plastic, and mason jars for salads (that's right, entire salads, Google it!).

→ Buy a measuring tape and, if you don't have one, a digital bathroom scale.

→ OPTIONAL: Buy the supplements you're going to use (if any).

→ OPTIONAL: Buy a pair of workout gloves if you want to protect your hands.

→ OPTIONAL: Buy a pair of squat shoes for better squatting and deadlifting.

→ OPTIONAL: Buy a pair of lasso straps for better pulling.

→ OPTIONAL: Buy a pair of shin guards or a few pairs of knee-high socks for bloodless (literally) deadlifting.

→ OPTIONAL: Buy equipment for your home gym.

2. JOIN OR SET UP A GYM

Many women are turned off by gyms, and understandably so.

Between the chorus of sweaty, smelly guys grunting, groaning, and gawking; the gaggles of wannabe Instagram celebrities busily snapping selfies; and the pack of stony-faced bodybuilders laying claim to every machine in the joint, there are plenty of reasons to feel about as comfortable in a gym as you would going for a swim in the Ohio River.

I want you to be able to tune all that out, though, and to see the gym through another lens—one I describe in my book *The Little Black Book of Workout Motivation* (www.workoutmotivation-book.com):

The gym is a lot more than a place to move, grunt, and sweat.

It's a microcosm where we can make contact with the deeper parts of ourselves—our convictions, fears, habits, and anxieties. It's an arena where we can confront these opponents head-on and prove we have what it takes to vanquish them.

It's a setting where we can test the stories we tell ourselves. It calls on us to demonstrate how we respond to the greater struggles of life—adversity, pain, insecurity, stress, weakness, and disadvantage—and, in some ways, who we really are. In this way, the gym is a training and testing ground for the body, mind, and soul.

The conflicts we learn to endure in the gym empower us in our daily lives as well. The concentration, discipline, and resilience carry over. The way to do anything is, at bottom, the way to do everything.

The gym is also a source of learning because it calls on us to constantly attempt new things. It's a forum where questions are at least as important as answers, and it cultivates what scientists call a "growth mindset" by teaching us that our abilities can be developed through dedication and hard work—a worldview that's essential for great accomplishment.

The gym is practical, too, not idealistic. It's a laboratory open to all ideas and methodologies, and it gives clear, unqualified feedback on them: either they work or they don't.

In short, the gym can be so much more than merely a place to work out. It can be a refuge from the chaos around us, a world of our own that we create to satisfy dreams and desires.

So, if you're on the fence about joining a gym, don't let yourself be talked or intimidated out of it. Take heart in the fact that you now know more than, well, probably everyone there, and before long, don't be surprised if people start coming to you for advice.

Plus, you have nothing to be self-conscious about. What many women don't realize about gyms is at least 90 percent of the people there are so intently focused on themselves that they give barely a glance to anyone around them.

So, assuming I've sold you on taking the plunge, the most important things to consider when picking a gym are:

1 Does it have the equipment you'll need to do your workouts?

Just about any gym that's well stocked with free weights and machines will do.

So long as it has a few bench presses and squat racks, a full set of dumbbells, and several basic machines—and allows deadlifting (important point!)—you're golden.

2 Is it close enough that you won't have any trouble going consistently?

I've found that if going to the gym requires more than about 40 minutes of total driving, compliance tends to suffer.

So, if you can, find a gym that's close to your home or office.

3 Does it fit your budget?

As with most things, you get what you pay for. Don't spend more on a gym than you can afford, but it's a good idea to invest a little money in going to one that's clean and has nice equipment, friendly staff, and other perks like showers, towels, cardio machines (if you want to do your cardio there), etc.

Most entry-level gym memberships will cost you anywhere from $10 to $50 per month, depending on where you live. Higher-tier gym memberships will cost anywhere from $100 to $300 per month.

For entry-level gyms, your best bets are going to be Gold's Gym, 24 Hour Fitness, LA Fitness, and Anytime Fitness. For premium gyms, Equinox and Life Time Fitness are great choices.

Your other option is a home gym, and this comes with pros and cons in terms of cost effectiveness, convenience, and privacy.

On the pro side:

→ You can't beat the convenience of working out in your own home, and this may make it easier to stick to the program.

→ You can train whenever you want and don't need to work around holiday hours or other schedule irregularities.

→ You never have to wait for someone to finish using equipment.

→ You can blare your favorite music, decorate the walls however you like, and more or less turn it into your own little fitness playground.

→ You save the time and money you'd have to spend commuting to and paying for a gym.

→ You don't have to worry about guys ogling you or sweating all over the equipment.

On the con side:

→ You're going to pay a couple thousand dollars for nice and new equipment, which doesn't include shipping or installation fees.

That's two years (give or take) of membership dues at a higher-end gym that costs $100 per month, like Equinox or Life Time Fitness.

→ You're going to be fairly limited in the exercises you can do, and if you want to do cardio on a machine, you'll need to buy that too.

→ You may enjoy your workouts less since you'll likely be alone while you train.

→ You have to maintain, repair, and replace your equipment.

→ You may get distracted by chores, kids, pets, your spouse or partner, etc.

Personally, I like to train at a commercial gym. It's slightly less convenient, but it allows me to do many different exercises, it helps me focus entirely on my training, I like meeting new people there, and I don't have to worry about waking up the kiddos when deadlifting.

That said, I do have a set of adjustable dumbbells and an exercise bike at home for whenever I want to sneak in some cardio and curls.

If you're going to be working out at home, then you need at least a few pieces of equipment. Here are the main ones:

→ Power Rack

A power rack, also called a squat rack, is a sturdy metal frame usually about eight feet tall, four feet wide, and three to six feet long with adjustable hooks to hold a barbell and safety bars to allow for safe solo weightlifting.

Many power racks also have pegs to hold weight plates.

This is what you'll use for the squat, bench press, pull-up, and chin-up.

→ Barbell

Many of the exercises in the program are going to require a barbell, so it's worth investing in a good one.

→ Weight Plates

You'll want to get at least two 2.5-, 5-, 10-, 25-, and 45-pound plates when you set up your home gym. You can buy more as you get stronger (most people like to add extra 10- and 45-pound plates).

Make sure you get round plates and not multi-sided ones, which shift out of position when you deadlift.

→ Adjustable Dumbbells

Adjustable dumbbells allow you to do just about any dumbbell exercise, and are much more space efficient than normal dumbbells.

→ Bench

You'll need a padded, adjustable bench with wheels that can be set completely flat or upright. This allows you to do your seated isolation exercises, and when combined with a power rack, allows you to do both flat and incline bench and dumbbell presses.

→ Deadlift Platform

A deadlift platform is a metal frame that sits on the ground and holds thick tiles of rubber.

As the name suggests, a deadlift platform allows you to deadlift without damaging the floor or your equipment or making too much noise.

It's also useful for barbell rowing for the same reasons.

You don't need a deadlift platform, but it'll let you descend faster while deadlifting and barbell rowing, which means you won't have to waste energy slowly lowering the weights.

You may want to add a dip station as well, which allows you to do both dips and leg raises.

There are countless other tools, toys, and machines you can buy, but you'll be able to do almost all the exercises in *Thinner Leaner Stronger* with this setup.

There are a few exercises you won't be able to do, like the lat pulldown, cable fly, seated cable row, and leg press, but you can substitute them for other "approved" exercises you can do. Simply go back to chapter 23 to find alternative exercises.

All told, you'll probably need $1,000 to $3,000 (depending on what type of equipment you want) and 100 to 200 square feet to put it together. For reference, the average two-car garage is 676 square feet.

In terms of where to set up your home gym, I recommend you pick a room that has a concrete floor, like a garage or unfinished basement.

I also recommend you set up your home gym on the first floor or in the basement because working out on an upper floor—and deadlifting in particular—can scare others in the house or even damage your floor.

3. TAKE YOUR FIRST MEASUREMENTS AND PICTURES

Remember the importance of taking measurements and pictures?

If you want a refresher, go back to chapter 31. Here's a summary of what you should do:

1. Take the following body measurements first thing in the morning, nude, after using the bathroom, and before eating or drinking anything:

   - Weight
   - Waist circumference
   - OPTIONAL: Hip circumference
   - OPTIONAL: Upper-leg circumference
   - OPTIONAL: Flexed arms

   Record your numbers in your phone, workout journal, or app, or somewhere else you prefer.

2. Take flexed and unflexed pictures from the front, back, and sides, and store them in an album or folder you can easily find.

   Remember to show as much skin as you feel comfortable with. The more the better because it'll give you the best idea of how your body is changing.

4. CREATE YOUR FIRST MEAL PLAN

You can go back to chapters 17 and 19 in *Thinner Leaner Stronger* if you want to do an in-depth review of how to calculate calories and macros and create a meal plan, but here's a simple check-list to get you through it:

1. Calculate your daily calorie target based on your goals.

2. Calculate your daily macronutrient targets based on your goals.

3. Load the meal-planning template in the free bonus material that comes with this book (www.thinnerleanerstronger.com/challengebonus), open up Excel or Google Sheets, or get a paper or notebook and pen.

4. Create a list of your preferred foods and recipes.

5. Familiarize yourself with the nutritional facts of your food choices using CalorieKing, SELF Nutrition Data, or the USDA Food Composition Databases.

6. Remove from your list any foods or recipes that are too high calorie or macronutritionally imbalanced to fit your needs.

7. Set up your pre- and postworkout meals first.

8. Add your primary sources of protein to the rest of your meals.

9. Add your fruits and vegetables.

10. Add any additional carbs and caloric beverages that aren't dessert or junk.

11. Tweak your protein intake as needed.

12. Add additional fat as needed.

13. Add treats if desired.

Remember that you want to be within 50 calories of your target intake when cutting and within 100 calories when lean bulking and maintaining.

5. CREATE YOUR WORKOUT SCHEDULE

Life is hectic and it always feels like there's never enough time in the 24 hours we get each day.

As I say in my book *The Little Black Book of Workout Motivation* (www.workoutmotivation-book.com):

Who has the time for half of all the stuff we want to do? I'm sorry that life isn't gift wrapping a chunk of your days so you can train in Zen-like comfort and solitude. Join the club. Face the fact that you're going to die with a long to-do list. Make damn sure "start training" isn't on that list.

What we're really talking about here is priorities. We have to make our fitness a top priority and only then will we be able to "find the time" to get our workouts in.

Thankfully, we don't need to find that much time to make it all work. As you'll recall from chapter 29, you have three *Thinner Leaner Stronger* workout routines to choose from:

1. A five-day routine
2. A four-day routine
3. A three-day routine

Each are weekly (seven-day) routines, so the most weightlifting you can do on the program is five workouts per week. Cardio isn't explicitly included in the routines because it's optional, and how much you do depends on how much time you have to give to it and whether you're cutting, lean bulking, or maintaining.

As far as results go, the five-day routine is better than the four- and three-day routines, and the four-day routine is better than the three-day routine. That doesn't mean you can't get great results with both the four- and three-day routines, though. You absolutely can.

So, decide now which routine you're going to follow, and then choose which days you're going to lift weights on. If you're going to do cardio workouts as well, decide how you want to fit those into your weekly schedule.

Here's what your week might look like if you were to do the five-day routine plus two cardio workouts:

- Monday: Lower Body (Legs and Glutes)
- Tuesday: Push and Core
- Wednesday: Pull and Cardio
- Thursday: Upper Body and Core
- Friday: Lower Body (Legs and Glutes)
- Saturday: Cardio
- Sunday: Rest

Here's what your week might look like if you were to do the four-day routine plus two cardio workouts:

- Monday: Lower Body (Legs and Glutes)
- Tuesday: Cardio
- Wednesday: Upper Body and Core
- Thursday: Pull
- Friday: Lower Body (Legs and Glutes)
- Saturday: Cardio
- Sunday: Rest

And here's what your week might look like if you were to do the three-day routine plus two cardio workouts:

- Monday: Lower Body (Legs and Glutes)
- Tuesday: Cardio
- Wednesday: Upper Body and Core
- Thursday: Cardio
- Friday: Lower Body and Pull (Legs and Back)
- Saturday: Rest
- Sunday: Rest

6. PREPARE FOR YOUR FIRST WEEK

1. Decide when to start *Thinner Leaner Stronger*.

   Mondays work best for most people as this leaves the weekend to prepare meals (if necessary).

2. Pick a day to prepare all your meals for your first week.

   If you want to learn more about effective meal prepping, go to:
   www.thinnerleanerstronger.com/mealprep.

3. Create a grocery list for everything you'll need to follow your meal plan for the first week, and then add any other items you need to buy.

4. Go grocery shopping. Buy what's on your list and nothing else.

5. OPTIONAL: Sort any snacks, treats, or calorie-dense foods you'll be tempted to overeat (nuts, dried fruit, chocolate, etc.) into smaller containers or bags.

6. Clean any tools or surfaces you'll need to prepare your meals (knives, countertops, pans, etc.).

7. Wash and chop all the foods you're going to cook.

8. Cook all your meals and store them in containers.

9. Make sure you have any supplements you're going to be taking.

10. Ensure you know exactly what you're supposed to do in your first week of workouts and that you have a way to track them (Excel or Google sheet, journal, app, or notepad).

11. Watch the form videos for all the exercises you're going to be doing in your first week, and practice the Big Three with a broomstick until you feel comfortable with the basic movements.

    Remember, links to videos showing proper form can be found in the free bonus material that comes with this book (www.thinnerleanerstronger.com/bonus).

You may want to save the PDF with links to these videos on your phone so you can pull them up in the gym as needed.

12. OPTIONAL: Announce on social media that you're starting Thinner Leaner Stronger, tag me (@muscleforlifefitness on Instagram and @muscleforlife on Twitter), and add the #thinner-leanerstronger hashtag.

13. OPTIONAL: Join my Facebook group and introduce yourself to this community of positive, supportive, like-minded people who are striving to become the best they can be.

You can find it at www.facebook.com/groups/muscleforlife.

7. DO YOUR FIRST WEEK

In chapter 29, you learned that week one is for finding your starting weights on all the exercises you'll be doing in your first training phase.

This is mostly a ma‑‑ter of trial and error. You start light on an exercise, try it out, and increase the weight for each successive hard set until you've dialed in everything.

You might find that the bar alone (45 pounds) feels quite heavy on some exercises (barbell squat, for instance) and may even be too heavy for others (bench press, for example).

Don't be discouraged by this. It's completely normal. You'll gain strength quickly, and before you know it, you'll be adding weight to the bar.

In cases where the bar is too much, you have two options:

1. You can switch to a dumbbell variation of the exercise until you're strong enough for the bar.

2. You can use a fixed-weight straight bar instead, which allows for less than 45 pounds.

For instance, if the bar is too heavy for the bench press (you can't get at least six to seven reps), you can do the dumbbell bench press instead or use a fixed bar lighter than 45 pounds.
You might also find your starting weights quickly and easily and feel comfortable diving right into proper hard sets in your first workouts. If that's the case, then be my guest!

As far as your diet goes, follow your meal and supplementation plans as closely as possible. Don't make on-the-fly food substitutions; try not to undereat, overeat, or eat "off-plan" foods or meals, treats, or even condiments; and take your supplements at the same time every day (so you don't forget and establish the habit).

Also, remember to weigh yourself daily so you can calculate your average daily weight at the end of the week.

8. GET READY FOR YOUR NEXT WEEK (AND BEYOND!)

With your first week in the books, it's time to congratulate yourself for work well done and prepare for the following week (and exciting journey ahead!).

That means adjusting your meal plan as needed, repeating your grocery shopping and meal prepping, taking new measurements and pictures, calculating your average daily weight for the previous week, and ensuring you have your next week's workouts penciled into your schedule.

Then, week after week, you simply repeat this routine, keeping a close eye on how your body is responding and modifying your diet and exercise accordingly.

And just like that, you're going to be on your way to the best shape of your life.

Keep eating, training, and supplementing according to everything you've learned in this book, and it won't be a matter of if but only when.

That's not all, either. If you're like the thousands of women I've spoken and worked with over the years, Thinner Leaner Stronger is going to give you a lot more than a new body. It's going to give you a new lease on life.

You're going to feel strong, sexy, and competent, and it's going to shine through in everything you do, both inside and outside the gym. People are going to start noticing and asking what the heck you're doing. You might not even believe the results yourself!

All that and more will be yours, and sooner rather than later.

POWER'S NOT GIVEN TO YOU. YOU HAVE TO TAKE IT.

—BEYONCÉ KNOWLES-CARTER

THINNER LEANER STRONGER PHASE 1

Lao Tzu famously said that the journey of a thousand miles begins with a single step, and I'm really excited that you're about to take YOUR first step in my program.

If you stick to the plan, you're going to see dramatic improvements in your body in just the next few months. People aren't going to believe their eyes. You might not either!

You're also going to enjoy the thrilling realization that you've finally discovered the "secret" to controlling your body composition, and that it's easier than you ever thought possible. Never again will you struggle to gain lean muscle or lose fat, and never again will you fall prey to mainstream diet and exercise fads and hucksters.

I have to warn you, though: the first 8 to 12 weeks are always the hardest.

I've worked with thousands of guys and gals over the years, and for whatever reason, if someone is going to quit, it's usually going to be within their first couple of months.

Sometimes it's because establishing new habits—even immediately beneficial ones—can be quite difficult, sometimes it's because they succumb to peer pressure to go back to their old unhealthy ways, and sometimes it's because of unforeseen disruptions like sickness, stress, or other shenanigans.

However, the people who can stick through the first two to three months, come hell or high water, often make it all the way. I want you to be one of these people. That's why I write books and articles, record podcasts and videos, and do everything else that I do.

So, can I ask a favor of you?

Can you promise me—and yourself—right now that you will do whatever it takes to get through the first two phases of this challenge?

You don't have to be perfect, of course—just good enough—and life may try to get in the way (in fact it probably will) and you may have to get creative to find work-arounds, but that's just part of the game.

The bottom line is this: if you make a firm decision to make it through, and then defend that decision no matter what comes, then there's nothing that can stop you.

So, are you ready?

Great. Let's begin by taking your first measurements and pictures.

First, take the following body measurements first thing in the morning, nude, after using the bathroom and before eating or drinking anything:

1. Weight
2. Waist circumference
3. OPTIONAL: Hip circumference
4. OPTIONAL: Upper-leg circumference
5. OPTIONAL: Flexed arms

Then, take flexed and unflexed pictures from the front, back, and sides, and store them in an album or folder that you can easily locate later.

Remember to show as much skin as you feel comfortable with. The more the better because it will give you the best idea of how your body is responding to the program.

On the following pages you'll find your first two months of hard training, followed by a deload week and new round of body measurements.

Oh, and if you haven't already, find me on social media and let me know how you're doing on the program! If you're going to post about it, be sure to include the #thinnerleanerstronger hashtag so that other people looking for Thinner Leaner Stronger inspiration will be able to find you and follow along.

———————

Here's how we can connect:
Facebook: www.facebook.com/muscleforlifefitness
Instagram: www.instagram.com/muscleforlifefitness
YouTube: www.youtube.com/muscleforlifefitness
Twitter: www.twitter.com/muscleforlife

That's it for now. Train hard and do well! I'll see you in two months!

5-DAY ROUTINE	PHASE 1	WEEK 1

WORKOUT 1: LOWER BODY (LEGS AND GLUTES)

EXERCISES	SETS		
Barbell Squat: Warm-up and 3 hard sets	×	×	×
Leg Press: 3 hard sets	×	×	×
Romanian Deadlift: 3 hard sets	×	×	×
Hip Thrust: 3 hard sets	×	×	×

NOTES:

WORKOUT 2: PUSH AND CORE

EXERCISES	SETS		
Barbell Bench Press: Warm-up and 3 hard sets	×	×	×
Seated Dumbbell Press: 3 hard sets	×	×	×
Dumbbell Bench Press: 3 hard sets	×	×	×
Dumbbell Side Lateral Raise: 3 hard sets	×	×	×
Crunch: 3 hard sets			

NOTES:

WORKOUT 3: PULL

EXERCISES	SETS		
Barbell Deadlift: Warm-up and 3 hard sets	×	×	×
One-Arm Dumbbell Row: 3 hard sets	×	×	×
Lat Pulldown (Wide-Grip): 3 hard sets	×	×	×
Barbell Curl: 3 hard sets	×	×	×

NOTES:

WORKOUT 4: UPPER BODY AND CORE			
EXERCISES	**SETS**		
Seated Dumbbell Press: Warm-up and 3 hard sets	×	×	×
Dumbbell Bench Press: 3 hard sets	×	×	×
Dumbbell Rear Lateral Raise (Seated): 3 hard sets	×	×	×
Seated Triceps Press: 3 hard sets	×	×	×
Captain's Chair Leg Raise: 3 hard sets			

NOTES:
_____
_____
_____

WORKOUT 5: LOWER BODY (LEGS AND GLUTES)			
EXERCISES	**SETS**		
Barbell Squat: Warm-up and 3 hard sets	×	×	×
Dumbbell Lunge (In-Place): 3 hard sets	×	×	×
Leg Curl (Lying or Seated)*: 3 hard sets	×	×	×
Glute Blaster: 3 hard sets	×	×	×

NOTES:
_____
_____
_____

5-DAY ROUTINE	PHASE 1	WEEK 2

WORKOUT 1: LOWER BODY (LEGS AND GLUTES)

EXERCISES	SETS		
Barbell Squat: Warm-up and 3 hard sets	×	×	×
Leg Press: 3 hard sets	×	×	×
Romanian Deadlift: 3 hard sets	×	×	×
Hip Thrust: 3 hard sets	×	×	×

NOTES:

WORKOUT 2: PUSH AND CORE

EXERCISES	SETS		
Barbell Bench Press: Warm-up and 3 hard sets	×	×	×
Seated Dumbbell Press: 3 hard sets	×	×	×
Dumbbell Bench Press: 3 hard sets	×	×	×
Dumbbell Side Lateral Raise: 3 hard sets	×	×	×
Crunch: 3 hard sets			

NOTES:

WORKOUT 3: PULL

EXERCISES	SETS		
Barbell Deadlift: Warm-up and 3 hard sets	×	×	×
One-Arm Dumbbell Row: 3 hard sets	×	×	×
Lat Pulldown (Wide-Grip): 3 hard sets	×	×	×
Barbell Curl: 3 hard sets	×	×	×

NOTES:

WORKOUT 4: UPPER BODY AND CORE			
EXERCISES	**SETS**		
Seated Dumbbell Press: Warm-up and 3 hard sets	×	×	×
Dumbbell Bench Press: 3 hard sets	×	×	×
Dumbbell Rear Lateral Raise (Seated): 3 hard sets	×	×	×
Seated Triceps Press: 3 hard sets	×	×	×
Captain's Chair Leg Raise: 3 hard sets			

NOTES:

_____

_____

_____

WORKOUT 5: LOWER BODY (LEGS AND GLUTES)			
EXERCISES	**SETS**		
Barbell Squat: Warm-up and 3 hard sets	×	×	×
Dumbbell Lunge (In-Place): 3 hard sets	×	×	×
Leg Curl (Lying or Seated)*: 3 hard sets	×	×	×
Glute Blaster: 3 hard sets	×	×	×

NOTES:

_____

_____

_____

5-DAY ROUTINE	PHASE 1	WEEK 3

WORKOUT 1: LOWER BODY (LEGS AND GLUTES)			
EXERCISES	SETS		
Barbell Squat: Warm-up and 3 hard sets	×	×	×
Leg Press: 3 hard sets	×	×	×
Romanian Deadlift: 3 hard sets	×	×	×
Hip Thrust: 3 hard sets	×	×	×

NOTES:

WORKOUT 2: PUSH AND CORE			
EXERCISES	SETS		
Barbell Bench Press: Warm-up and 3 hard sets	×	×	×
Seated Dumbbell Press: 3 hard sets	×	×	×
Dumbbell Bench Press: 3 hard sets	×	×	×
Dumbbell Side Lateral Raise: 3 hard sets	×	×	×
Crunch: 3 hard sets			

NOTES:

WORKOUT 3: PULL			
EXERCISES	SETS		
Barbell Deadlift: Warm-up and 3 hard sets	×	×	×
One-Arm Dumbbell Row: 3 hard sets	×	×	×
Lat Pulldown (Wide-Grip): 3 hard sets	×	×	×
Barbell Curl: 3 hard sets	×	×	×

NOTES:

WORKOUT 4: UPPER BODY AND CORE			
EXERCISES	SETS		
Seated Dumbbell Press: Warm-up and 3 hard sets	×	×	×
Dumbbell Bench Press: 3 hard sets	×	×	×
Dumbbell Rear Lateral Raise (Seated): 3 hard sets	×	×	×
Seated Triceps Press: 3 hard sets	×	×	×
Captain's Chair Leg Raise: 3 hard sets			

NOTES:

WORKOUT 5: LOWER BODY (LEGS AND GLUTES)			
EXERCISES	SETS		
Barbell Squat: Warm-up and 3 hard sets	×	×	×
Dumbbell Lunge (In-Place): 3 hard sets	×	×	×
Leg Curl (Lying or Seated)*: 3 hard sets	×	×	×
Glute Blaster: 3 hard sets	×	×	×

NOTES:

5-DAY ROUTINE	PHASE 1	WEEK 4

WORKOUT 1: LOWER BODY (LEGS AND GLUTES)

EXERCISES	SETS		
Barbell Squat: Warm-up and 3 hard sets	×	×	×
Leg Press: 3 hard sets	×	×	×
Romanian Deadlift: 3 hard sets	×	×	×
Hip Thrust: 3 hard sets	×	×	×

NOTES:

_____

_____

_____

WORKOUT 2: PUSH AND CORE

EXERCISES	SETS		
Barbell Bench Press: Warm-up and 3 hard sets	×	×	×
Seated Dumbbell Press: 3 hard sets	×	×	×
Dumbbell Bench Press: 3 hard sets	×	×	×
Dumbbell Side Lateral Raise: 3 hard sets	×	×	×
Crunch: 3 hard sets			

NOTES:

_____

_____

_____

WORKOUT 3: PULL

EXERCISES	SETS		
Barbell Deadlift: Warm-up and 3 hard sets	×	×	×
One-Arm Dumbbell Row: 3 hard sets	×	×	×
Lat Pulldown (Wide-Grip): 3 hard sets	×	×	×
Barbell Curl: 3 hard sets	×	×	×

NOTES:

_____

_____

_____

WORKOUT 4: UPPER BODY AND CORE			
EXERCISES	SETS		
Seated Dumbbell Press: Warm-up and 3 hard sets	×	×	×
Dumbbell Bench Press: 3 hard sets	×	×	×
Dumbbell Rear Lateral Raise (Seated): 3 hard sets	×	×	×
Seated Triceps Press: 3 hard sets	×	×	×
Captain's Chair Leg Raise: 3 hard sets			

NOTES:

WORKOUT 5: LOWER BODY (LEGS AND GLUTES)			
EXERCISES	SETS		
Barbell Squat: Warm-up and 3 hard sets	×	×	×
Dumbbell Lunge (In-Place): 3 hard sets	×	×	×
Leg Curl (Lying or Seated)*: 3 hard sets	×	×	×
Glute Blaster: 3 hard sets	×	×	×

NOTES:

5-DAY ROUTINE | PHASE 1 | WEEK 5

WORKOUT 1: LOWER BODY (LEGS AND GLUTES)

EXERCISES	SETS		
Barbell Squat: Warm-up and 3 hard sets	×	×	×
Leg Press: 3 hard sets	×	×	×
Romanian Deadlift: 3 hard sets	×	×	×
Hip Thrust: 3 hard sets	×	×	×

NOTES:

WORKOUT 2: PUSH AND CORE

EXERCISES	SETS		
Barbell Bench Press: Warm-up and 3 hard sets	×	×	×
Seated Dumbbell Press: 3 hard sets	×	×	×
Dumbbell Bench Press: 3 hard sets	×	×	×
Dumbbell Side Lateral Raise: 3 hard sets	×	×	×
Crunch: 3 hard sets			

NOTES:

WORKOUT 3: PULL

EXERCISES	SETS		
Barbell Deadlift: Warm-up and 3 hard sets	×	×	×
One-Arm Dumbbell Row: 3 hard sets	×	×	×
Lat Pulldown (Wide-Grip): 3 hard sets	×	×	×
Barbell Curl: 3 hard sets	×	×	×

NOTES:

WORKOUT 4: UPPER BODY AND CORE			
EXERCISES	**SETS**		
Seated Dumbbell Press: Warm-up and 3 hard sets	×	×	×
Dumbbell Bench Press: 3 hard sets	×	×	×
Dumbbell Rear Lateral Raise (Seated): 3 hard sets	×	×	×
Seated Triceps Press: 3 hard sets	×	×	×
Captain's Chair Leg Raise: 3 hard sets			

NOTES:

_____

_____

_____

WORKOUT 5: LOWER BODY (LEGS AND GLUTES)			
EXERCISES	**SETS**		
Barbell Squat: Warm-up and 3 hard sets	×	×	×
Dumbbell Lunge (In-Place): 3 hard sets	×	×	×
Leg Curl (Lying or Seated)*: 3 hard sets	×	×	×
Glute Blaster: 3 hard sets	×	×	×

NOTES:

_____

_____

_____

5-DAY ROUTINE | PHASE 1 | WEEK 6

WORKOUT 1: LOWER BODY (LEGS AND GLUTES)

EXERCISES	SETS		
Barbell Squat: Warm-up and 3 hard sets	×	×	×
Leg Press: 3 hard sets	×	×	×
Romanian Deadlift: 3 hard sets	×	×	×
Hip Thrust: 3 hard sets	×	×	×

NOTES:

WORKOUT 2: PUSH AND CORE

EXERCISES	SETS		
Barbell Bench Press: Warm-up and 3 hard sets	×	×	×
Seated Dumbbell Press: 3 hard sets	×	×	×
Dumbbell Bench Press: 3 hard sets	×	×	×
Dumbbell Side Lateral Raise: 3 hard sets	×	×	×
Crunch: 3 hard sets			

NOTES:

WORKOUT 3: PULL

EXERCISES	SETS		
Barbell Deadlift: Warm-up and 3 hard sets	×	×	×
One-Arm Dumbbell Row: 3 hard sets	×	×	×
Lat Pulldown (Wide-Grip): 3 hard sets	×	×	×
Barbell Curl: 3 hard sets	×	×	×

NOTES:

WORKOUT 4: UPPER BODY AND CORE			
EXERCISES	**SETS**		
Seated Dumbbell Press: Warm-up and 3 hard sets	×	×	×
Dumbbell Bench Press: 3 hard sets	×	×	×
Dumbbell Rear Lateral Raise (Seated): 3 hard sets	×	×	×
Seated Triceps Press: 3 hard sets	×	×	×
Captain's Chair Leg Raise: 3 hard sets			

NOTES:

_____

_____

_____

WORKOUT 5: LOWER BODY (LEGS AND GLUTES)			
EXERCISES	**SETS**		
Barbell Squat: Warm-up and 3 hard sets	×	×	×
Dumbbell Lunge (In-Place): 3 hard sets	×	×	×
Leg Curl (Lying or Seated)*: 3 hard sets	×	×	×
Glute Blaster: 3 hard sets	×	×	×

NOTES:

_____

_____

_____

| 5-DAY ROUTINE | PHASE 1 | WEEK 7 |

WORKOUT 1: LOWER BODY (LEGS AND GLUTES)

EXERCISES	SETS		
Barbell Squat: Warm-up and 3 hard sets	×	×	×
Leg Press: 3 hard sets	×	×	×
Romanian Deadlift: 3 hard sets	×	×	×
Hip Thrust: 3 hard sets	×	×	×

NOTES:

WORKOUT 2: PUSH AND CORE

EXERCISES	SETS		
Barbell Bench Press: Warm-up and 3 hard sets	×	×	×
Seated Dumbbell Press: 3 hard sets	×	×	×
Dumbbell Bench Press: 3 hard sets	×	×	×
Dumbbell Side Lateral Raise: 3 hard sets	×	×	×
Crunch: 3 hard sets			

NOTES:

WORKOUT 3: PULL

EXERCISES	SETS		
Barbell Deadlift: Warm-up and 3 hard sets	×	×	×
One-Arm Dumbbell Row: 3 hard sets	×	×	×
Lat Pulldown (Wide-Grip): 3 hard sets	×	×	×
Barbell Curl: 3 hard sets	×	×	×

NOTES:

WORKOUT 4: UPPER BODY AND CORE			
EXERCISES	SETS		
Seated Dumbbell Press: Warm-up and 3 hard sets	×	×	×
Dumbbell Bench Press: 3 hard sets	×	×	×
Dumbbell Rear Lateral Raise (Seated): 3 hard sets	×	×	×
Seated Triceps Press: 3 hard sets	×	×	×
Captain's Chair Leg Raise: 3 hard sets			

NOTES:

WORKOUT 5: LOWER BODY (LEGS AND GLUTES)			
EXERCISES	SETS		
Barbell Squat: Warm-up and 3 hard sets	×	×	×
Dumbbell Lunge (In-Place): 3 hard sets	×	×	×
Leg Curl (Lying or Seated)*: 3 hard sets	×	×	×
Glute Blaster: 3 hard sets	×	×	×

NOTES:

5-DAY ROUTINE | PHASE 1 | WEEK 8

WORKOUT 1: LOWER BODY (LEGS AND GLUTES)

EXERCISES	SETS		
Barbell Squat: Warm-up and 3 hard sets	×	×	×
Leg Press: 3 hard sets	×	×	×
Romanian Deadlift: 3 hard sets	×	×	×
Hip Thrust: 3 hard sets	×	×	×

NOTES:

WORKOUT 2: PUSH AND CORE

EXERCISES	SETS		
Barbell Bench Press: Warm-up and 3 hard sets	×	×	×
Seated Dumbbell Press: 3 hard sets	×	×	×
Dumbbell Bench Press: 3 hard sets	×	×	×
Dumbbell Side Lateral Raise: 3 hard sets	×	×	×
Crunch: 3 hard sets			

NOTES:

WORKOUT 3: PULL

EXERCISES	SETS		
Barbell Deadlift: Warm-up and 3 hard sets	×	×	×
One-Arm Dumbbell Row: 3 hard sets	×	×	×
Lat Pulldown (Wide-Grip): 3 hard sets	×	×	×
Barbell Curl: 3 hard sets	×	×	×

NOTES:

WORKOUT 4: UPPER BODY AND CORE			
EXERCISES	**SETS**		
Seated Dumbbell Press: Warm-up and 3 hard sets	×	×	×
Dumbbell Bench Press: 3 hard sets	×	×	×
Dumbbell Rear Lateral Raise (Seated): 3 hard sets	×	×	×
Seated Triceps Press: 3 hard sets	×	×	×
Captain's Chair Leg Raise: 3 hard sets			

NOTES:

WORKOUT 5: LOWER BODY (LEGS AND GLUTES)			
EXERCISES	**SETS**		
Barbell Squat: Warm-up and 3 hard sets	×	×	×
Dumbbell Lunge (In-Place): 3 hard sets	×	×	×
Leg Curl (Lying or Seated)*: 3 hard sets	×	×	×
Glute Blaster: 3 hard sets	×	×	×

NOTES:

| 5-DAY ROUTINE | DELOAD | WEEK 9 |

WORKOUT 1: DELOAD LEGS

EXERCISES	SETS		
Barbell Squat: Warm-up and 3 sets of 5 reps with last hard set weight	×	×	×
Romanian Deadlift: 3 sets of 5 reps with last hard set weight	×	×	×
Hip Thrust: 3 sets of 5 reps with last hard set weight	×	×	×

NOTES: _____

_____

WORKOUT 2: DELOAD PUSH

EXERCISES	SETS		
Barbell Bench Press: Warm-up and 3 sets of 5 reps with last hard set weight	×	×	×
Seated Dumbbell Press: 3 sets of 5 reps with last hard set weight	×	×	×
Dumbbell Side Lateral Raise: 3 sets of 5 reps with last hard set weight	×	×	×

NOTES: _____

_____

WORKOUT 3: DELOAD PULL

EXERCISES	SETS		
Barbell Deadlift: Warm-up and 3 sets of 5 reps with last hard set weight	×	×	×
Barbell Row: 3 sets of 5 reps with last hard set weight	×	×	×
Lat Pulldown (Wide-Grip): 3 sets of 5 reps with last hard set weight	×	×	×

NOTES: _____

_____

4-DAY ROUTINE	PHASE 1	WEEK 1

WORKOUT 1: LOWER BODY (LEGS AND GLUTES)			
EXERCISES	**SETS**		
Barbell Squat: Warm-up and 3 hard sets	×	×	×
Leg Press: 3 hard sets	×	×	×
Romanian Deadlift: 3 hard sets	×	×	×
Hip Thrust: 3 hard sets	×	×	×

NOTES:

WORKOUT 2: UPPER BODY AND CORE			
EXERCISES	**SETS**		
Barbell Bench Press: Warm-up and 3 hard sets	×	×	×
Seated Dumbbell Press: 3 hard sets	×	×	×
Dumbbell Side Lateral Raise: 3 hard sets	×	×	×
Seated Triceps Press: 3 hard sets	×	×	×
Crunch: 3 hard sets			

NOTES:

WORKOUT 3: PULL			
EXERCISES	**SETS**		
Barbell Deadlift: Warm-up and 3 hard sets	×	×	×
One-Arm Dumbbell Row: 3 hard sets	×	×	×
Lat Pulldown (Wide-Grip): 3 hard sets	×	×	×
Barbell Curl: 3 hard sets	×	×	×

NOTES:

_____

_____

_____

WORKOUT 4: LOWER BODY (LEGS AND GLUTES)			
EXERCISES	**SETS**		
Barbell Squat: Warm-up and 3 hard sets	×	×	×
Dumbbell Lunge (In-Place): 3 hard sets	×	×	×
Leg Curl (Lying or Seated)*: 3 hard sets	×	×	×
Glute Blaster: 3 hard sets	×	×	×

NOTES:

_____

_____

_____

4-DAY ROUTINE	PHASE 1	WEEK 2

WORKOUT 1: LOWER BODY (LEGS AND GLUTES)			
EXERCISES	**SETS**		
Barbell Squat: Warm-up and 3 hard sets	×	×	×
Leg Press: 3 hard sets	×	×	×
Romanian Deadlift: 3 hard sets	×	×	×
Hip Thrust: 3 hard sets	×	×	×

NOTES:

WORKOUT 2: UPPER BODY AND CORE			
EXERCISES	**SETS**		
Barbell Bench Press: Warm-up and 3 hard sets	×	×	×
Seated Dumbbell Press: 3 hard sets	×	×	×
Dumbbell Side Lateral Raise: 3 hard sets	×	×	×
Seated Triceps Press: 3 hard sets	×	×	×
Crunch: 3 hard sets			

NOTES:

WORKOUT 3: PULL			
EXERCISES	**SETS**		
Barbell Deadlift: Warm-up and 3 hard sets	×	×	×
One-Arm Dumbbell Row: 3 hard sets	×	×	×
Lat Pulldown (Wide-Grip): 3 hard sets	×	×	×
Barbell Curl: 3 hard sets	×	×	×

NOTES:

_____

_____

_____

WORKOUT 4: LOWER BODY (LEGS AND GLUTES)			
EXERCISES	**SETS**		
Barbell Squat: Warm-up and 3 hard sets	×	×	×
Dumbbell Lunge (In-Place): 3 hard sets	×	×	×
Leg Curl (Lying or Seated)*: 3 hard sets	×	×	×
Glute Blaster: 3 hard sets	×	×	×

NOTES:

_____

_____

_____

4-DAY ROUTINE	PHASE 1	WEEK 3

WORKOUT 1: LOWER BODY (LEGS AND GLUTES)			
EXERCISES	**SETS**		
Barbell Squat: Warm-up and 3 hard sets	×	×	×
Leg Press: 3 hard sets	×	×	×
Romanian Deadlift: 3 hard sets	×	×	×
Hip Thrust: 3 hard sets	×	×	×

NOTES:

WORKOUT 2: UPPER BODY AND CORE			
EXERCISES	**SETS**		
Barbell Bench Press: Warm-up and 3 hard sets	×	×	×
Seated Dumbbell Press: 3 hard sets	×	×	×
Dumbbell Side Lateral Raise: 3 hard sets	×	×	×
Seated Triceps Press: 3 hard sets	×	×	×
Crunch: 3 hard sets			

NOTES:

THE YEAR ONE CHALLENGE FOR WOMEN **107**

WORKOUT 3: PULL			
EXERCISES	**SETS**		
Barbell Deadlift: Warm-up and 3 hard sets	×	×	×
One-Arm Dumbbell Row: 3 hard sets	×	×	×
Lat Pulldown (Wide-Grip): 3 hard sets	×	×	×
Barbell Curl: 3 hard sets	×	×	×

NOTES:

_____

_____

_____

WORKOUT 4: LOWER BODY (LEGS AND GLUTES)			
EXERCISES	**SETS**		
Barbell Squat: Warm-up and 3 hard sets	×	×	×
Dumbbell Lunge (In-Place): 3 hard sets	×	×	×
Leg Curl (Lying or Seated)*: 3 hard sets	×	×	×
Glute Blaster: 3 hard sets	×	×	×

NOTES:

_____

_____

_____

4-DAY ROUTINE	PHASE 1	WEEK 4

WORKOUT 1: LOWER BODY (LEGS AND GLUTES)			
EXERCISES	**SETS**		
Barbell Squat: Warm-up and 3 hard sets	×	×	×
Leg Press: 3 hard sets	×	×	×
Romanian Deadlift: 3 hard sets	×	×	×
Hip Thrust: 3 hard sets	×	×	×

NOTES:

WORKOUT 2: UPPER BODY AND CORE			
EXERCISES	**SETS**		
Barbell Bench Press: Warm-up and 3 hard sets	×	×	×
Seated Dumbbell Press: 3 hard sets	×	×	×
Dumbbell Side Lateral Raise: 3 hard sets	×	×	×
Seated Triceps Press: 3 hard sets	×	×	×
Crunch: 3 hard sets			

NOTES:

WORKOUT 3: PULL			
EXERCISES	**SETS**		
Barbell Deadlift: Warm-up and 3 hard sets	×	×	×
One-Arm Dumbbell Row: 3 hard sets	×	×	×
Lat Pulldown (Wide-Grip): 3 hard sets	×	×	×
Barbell Curl: 3 hard sets	×	×	×

NOTES:

_____

_____

_____

WORKOUT 4: LOWER BODY (LEGS AND GLUTES)			
EXERCISES	**SETS**		
Barbell Squat: Warm-up and 3 hard sets	×	×	×
Dumbbell Lunge (In-Place): 3 hard sets	×	×	×
Leg Curl (Lying or Seated)*: 3 hard sets	×	×	×
Glute Blaster: 3 hard sets	×	×	×

NOTES:

_____

_____

_____

4-DAY ROUTINE	PHASE 1	WEEK 5

WORKOUT 1: LOWER BODY (LEGS AND GLUTES)			
EXERCISES	**SETS**		
Barbell Squat: Warm-up and 3 hard sets	×	×	×
Leg Press: 3 hard sets	×	×	×
Romanian Deadlift: 3 hard sets	×	×	×
Hip Thrust: 3 hard sets	×	×	×

NOTES:

WORKOUT 2: UPPER BODY AND CORE			
EXERCISES	**SETS**		
Barbell Bench Press: Warm-up and 3 hard sets	×	×	×
Seated Dumbbell Press: 3 hard sets	×	×	×
Dumbbell Side Lateral Raise: 3 hard sets	×	×	×
Seated Triceps Press: 3 hard sets	×	×	×
Crunch: 3 hard sets			

NOTES:

WORKOUT 3: PULL			
EXERCISES	**SETS**		
Barbell Deadlift: Warm-up and 3 hard sets	×	×	×
One-Arm Dumbbell Row: 3 hard sets	×	×	×
Lat Pulldown (Wide-Grip): 3 hard sets	×	×	×
Barbell Curl: 3 hard sets	×	×	×

NOTES:
_____
_____
_____

WORKOUT 4: LOWER BODY (LEGS AND GLUTES)			
EXERCISES	**SETS**		
Barbell Squat: Warm-up and 3 hard sets	×	×	×
Dumbbell Lunge (In-Place): 3 hard sets	×	×	×
Leg Curl (Lying or Seated)*: 3 hard sets	×	×	×
Glute Blaster: 3 hard sets	×	×	×

NOTES:
_____
_____
_____

4-DAY ROUTINE	PHASE 1	WEEK 6

WORKOUT 1: LOWER BODY (LEGS AND GLUTES)			
EXERCISES	**SETS**		
Barbell Squat: Warm-up and 3 hard sets	×	×	×
Leg Press: 3 hard sets	×	×	×
Romanian Deadlift: 3 hard sets	×	×	×
Hip Thrust: 3 hard sets	×	×	×

NOTES:

_____

_____

_____

WORKOUT 2: UPPER BODY AND CORE			
EXERCISES	**SETS**		
Barbell Bench Press: Warm-up and 3 hard sets	×	×	×
Seated Dumbbell Press: 3 hard sets	×	×	×
Dumbbell Side Lateral Raise: 3 hard sets	×	×	×
Seated Triceps Press: 3 hard sets	×	×	×
Crunch: 3 hard sets			

NOTES:

_____

_____

_____

WORKOUT 3: PULL			
EXERCISES	**SETS**		
Barbell Deadlift: Warm-up and 3 hard sets	×	×	×
One-Arm Dumbbell Row: 3 hard sets	×	×	×
Lat Pulldown (Wide-Grip): 3 hard sets	×	×	×
Barbell Curl: 3 hard sets	×	×	×

NOTES:

_____

_____

_____

WORKOUT 4: LOWER BODY (LEGS AND GLUTES)			
EXERCISES	**SETS**		
Barbell Squat: Warm-up and 3 hard sets	×	×	×
Dumbbell Lunge (In-Place): 3 hard sets	×	×	×
Leg Curl (Lying or Seated)*: 3 hard sets	×	×	×
Glute Blaster: 3 hard sets	×	×	×

NOTES:

_____

_____

_____

4-DAY ROUTINE	PHASE 1	WEEK 7

WORKOUT 1: LOWER BODY (LEGS AND GLUTES)			
EXERCISES	**SETS**		
Barbell Squat: Warm-up and 3 hard sets	×	×	×
Leg Press: 3 hard sets	×	×	×
Romanian Deadlift: 3 hard sets	×	×	×
Hip Thrust: 3 hard sets	×	×	×

NOTES:

WORKOUT 2: UPPER BODY AND CORE			
EXERCISES	**SETS**		
Barbell Bench Press: Warm-up and 3 hard sets	×	×	×
Seated Dumbbell Press: 3 hard sets	×	×	×
Dumbbell Side Lateral Raise: 3 hard sets	×	×	×
Seated Triceps Press: 3 hard sets	×	×	×
Crunch: 3 hard sets			

NOTES:

WORKOUT 3: PULL			
EXERCISES	**SETS**		
Barbell Deadlift: Warm-up and 3 hard sets	×	×	×
One-Arm Dumbbell Row: 3 hard sets	×	×	×
Lat Pulldown (Wide-Grip): 3 hard sets	×	×	×
Barbell Curl: 3 hard sets	×	×	×

NOTES:

_____

_____

_____

WORKOUT 4: LOWER BODY (LEGS AND GLUTES)			
EXERCISES	**SETS**		
Barbell Squat: Warm-up and 3 hard sets	×	×	×
Dumbbell Lunge (In-Place): 3 hard sets	×	×	×
Leg Curl (Lying or Seated)*: 3 hard sets	×	×	×
Glute Blaster: 3 hard sets	×	×	×

NOTES:

_____

_____

_____

4-DAY ROUTINE	PHASE 1	WEEK 8

WORKOUT 1: LOWER BODY (LEGS AND GLUTES)			
EXERCISES	**SETS**		
Barbell Squat: Warm-up and 3 hard sets	×	×	×
Leg Press: 3 hard sets	×	×	×
Romanian Deadlift: 3 hard sets	×	×	×
Hip Thrust: 3 hard sets	×	×	×

NOTES:

_____

_____

WORKOUT 2: UPPER BODY AND CORE			
EXERCISES	**SETS**		
Barbell Bench Press: Warm-up and 3 hard sets	×	×	×
Seated Dumbbell Press: 3 hard sets	×	×	×
Dumbbell Side Lateral Raise: 3 hard sets	×	×	×
Seated Triceps Press: 3 hard sets	×	×	×
Crunch: 3 hard sets			

NOTES:

_____

_____

WORKOUT 3: PULL			
EXERCISES	**SETS**		
Barbell Deadlift: Warm-up and 3 hard sets	×	×	×
One-Arm Dumbbell Row: 3 hard sets	×	×	×
Lat Pulldown (Wide-Grip): 3 hard sets	×	×	×
Barbell Curl: 3 hard sets	×	×	×

NOTES:
_____
_____
_____

WORKOUT 4: LOWER BODY (LEGS AND GLUTES)			
EXERCISES	**SETS**		
Barbell Squat: Warm-up and 3 hard sets	×	×	×
Dumbbell Lunge (In-Place): 3 hard sets	×	×	×
Leg Curl (Lying or Seated)*: 3 hard sets	×	×	×
Glute Blaster: 3 hard sets	×	×	×

NOTES:
_____
_____
_____

| 4-DAY ROUTINE | DELOAD | WEEK 9 |

WORKOUT 1: DELOAD LEGS

EXERCISES	SETS		
Barbell Squat: Warm-up and 3 sets of 5 reps with last hard set weight	×	×	×
Romanian Deadlift: 3 sets of 5 reps with last hard set weight	×	×	×
Hip Thrust: 3 sets of 5 reps with last hard set weight	×	×	×

NOTES:

_____

_____

_____

WORKOUT 2: DELOAD PUSH

EXERCISES	SETS		
Barbell Bench Press: Warm-up and 3 sets of 5 reps with last hard set weight	×	×	×
Seated Dumbbell Press: 3 sets of 5 reps with last hard set weight	×	×	×
Dumbbell Bench Press: 3 sets of 5 reps with last hard set weight	×	×	×

NOTES:

_____

_____

_____

WORKOUT 3: DELOAD PULL

EXERCISES	SETS		
Barbell Deadlift: Warm-up and 3 sets of 5 reps with last hard set weight	×	×	×
Barbell Row: 3 sets of 5 reps with last hard set weight	×	×	×
Lat Pulldown (Wide-Grip): 3 sets of 5 reps with last hard set weight	×	×	×

NOTES:

_____

_____

_____

| 3-DAY ROUTINE | PHASE 1 | WEEK 1 |

WORKOUT 1: LOWER BODY (LEGS AND GLUTES)

EXERCISES	SETS		
Barbell Squat: Warm-up and 3 hard sets	×	×	×
Leg Press: 3 hard sets	×	×	×
Romanian Deadlift: 3 hard sets	×	×	×
Hip Thrust: 3 hard sets	×	×	×

NOTES:

WORKOUT 2: UPPER BODY AND CORE

EXERCISES	SETS		
Barbell Bench Press: Warm-up and 3 hard sets	×	×	×
Seated Dumbbell Press: 3 hard sets	×	×	×
Dumbbell Side Lateral Raise: 3 hard sets	×	×	×
Seated Triceps Press: 3 hard sets	×	×	×
Crunch: 3 hard sets			

NOTES:

WORKOUT 3: LOWER BODY AND PULL (LEGS AND BACK)

EXERCISES	SETS		
Barbell Squat: Warm-up and 3 hard sets	×	×	×
Barbell Deadlift: Warm-up and 3 hard sets	×	×	×
One-Arm Dumbbell Row: 3 hard sets	×	×	×
Lat Pulldown (Wide-Grip): 3 hard sets	×	×	×
Barbell Curl: 3 hard sets	×	×	×

NOTES:

3-DAY ROUTINE	PHASE 1	WEEK 2

WORKOUT 1: LOWER BODY (LEGS AND GLUTES)			
EXERCISES	**SETS**		
Barbell Squat: Warm-up and 3 hard sets	×	×	×
Leg Press: 3 hard sets	×	×	×
Romanian Deadlift: 3 hard sets	×	×	×
Hip Thrust: 3 hard sets	×	×	×

NOTES:

WORKOUT 2: UPPER BODY AND CORE			
EXERCISES	**SETS**		
Barbell Bench Press: Warm-up and 3 hard sets	×	×	×
Seated Dumbbell Press: 3 hard sets	×	×	×
Dumbbell Side Lateral Raise: 3 hard sets	×	×	×
Seated Triceps Press: 3 hard sets	×	×	×
Crunch: 3 hard sets			

NOTES:

WORKOUT 3: LOWER BODY AND PULL (LEGS AND BACK)			
EXERCISES	**SETS**		
Barbell Squat: Warm-up and 3 hard sets	×	×	×
Barbell Deadlift: Warm-up and 3 hard sets	×	×	×
One-Arm Dumbbell Row: 3 hard sets	×	×	×
Lat Pulldown (Wide-Grip): 3 hard sets	×	×	×
Barbell Curl: 3 hard sets	×	×	×

NOTES:

3-DAY ROUTINE | PHASE 1 | WEEK 3

WORKOUT 1: LOWER BODY (LEGS AND GLUTES)

EXERCISES	SETS		
Barbell Squat: Warm-up and 3 hard sets	×	×	×
Leg Press: 3 hard sets	×	×	×
Romanian Deadlift: 3 hard sets	×	×	×
Hip Thrust: 3 hard sets	×	×	×

NOTES:

WORKOUT 2: UPPER BODY AND CORE

EXERCISES	SETS		
Barbell Bench Press: Warm-up and 3 hard sets	×	×	×
Seated Dumbbell Press: 3 hard sets	×	×	×
Dumbbell Side Lateral Raise: 3 hard sets	×	×	×
Seated Triceps Press: 3 hard sets	×	×	×
Crunch: 3 hard sets			

NOTES:

WORKOUT 3: LOWER BODY AND PULL (LEGS AND BACK)

EXERCISES	SETS		
Barbell Squat: Warm-up and 3 hard sets	×	×	×
Barbell Deadlift: Warm-up and 3 hard sets	×	×	×
One-Arm Dumbbell Row: 3 hard sets	×	×	×
Lat Pulldown (Wide-Grip): 3 hard sets	×	×	×
Barbell Curl: 3 hard sets	×	×	×

NOTES:

| 3-DAY ROUTINE | PHASE 1 | WEEK 4 |

WORKOUT 1: LOWER BODY (LEGS AND GLUTES)

EXERCISES	SETS		
Barbell Squat: Warm-up and 3 hard sets	×	×	×
Leg Press: 3 hard sets	×	×	×
Romanian Deadlift: 3 hard sets	×	×	×
Hip Thrust: 3 hard sets	×	×	×

NOTES:

WORKOUT 2: UPPER BODY AND CORE

EXERCISES	SETS		
Barbell Bench Press: Warm-up and 3 hard sets	×	×	×
Seated Dumbbell Press: 3 hard sets	×	×	×
Dumbbell Side Lateral Raise: 3 hard sets	×	×	×
Seated Triceps Press: 3 hard sets	×	×	×
Crunch: 3 hard sets			

NOTES:

WORKOUT 3: LOWER BODY AND PULL (LEGS AND BACK)

EXERCISES	SETS		
Barbell Squat: Warm-up and 3 hard sets	×	×	×
Barbell Deadlift: Warm-up and 3 hard sets	×	×	×
One-Arm Dumbbell Row: 3 hard sets	×	×	×
Lat Pulldown (Wide-Grip): 3 hard sets	×	×	×
Barbell Curl: 3 hard sets	×	×	×

NOTES:

3-DAY ROUTINE | PHASE 1 | WEEK 5

WORKOUT 1: LOWER BODY (LEGS AND GLUTES)

EXERCISES	SETS		
Barbell Squat: Warm-up and 3 hard sets	×	×	×
Leg Press: 3 hard sets	×	×	×
Romanian Deadlift: 3 hard sets	×	×	×
Hip Thrust: 3 hard sets	×	×	×

NOTES:

WORKOUT 2: UPPER BODY AND CORE

EXERCISES	SETS		
Barbell Bench Press: Warm-up and 3 hard sets	×	×	×
Seated Dumbbell Press: 3 hard sets	×	×	×
Dumbbell Side Lateral Raise: 3 hard sets	×	×	×
Seated Triceps Press: 3 hard sets	×	×	×
Crunch: 3 hard sets			

NOTES:

WORKOUT 3: LOWER BODY AND PULL (LEGS AND BACK)

EXERCISES	SETS		
Barbell Squat: Warm-up and 3 hard sets	×	×	×
Barbell Deadlift: Warm-up and 3 hard sets	×	×	×
One-Arm Dumbbell Row: 3 hard sets	×	×	×
Lat Pulldown (Wide-Grip): 3 hard sets	×	×	×
Barbell Curl: 3 hard sets	×	×	×

NOTES:

3-DAY ROUTINE	PHASE 1	WEEK 6

WORKOUT 1: LOWER BODY (LEGS AND GLUTES)

EXERCISES	SETS		
Barbell Squat: Warm-up and 3 hard sets	×	×	×
Leg Press: 3 hard sets	×	×	×
Romanian Deadlift: 3 hard sets	×	×	×
Hip Thrust: 3 hard sets	×	×	×

NOTES:

WORKOUT 2: UPPER BODY AND CORE

EXERCISES	SETS		
Barbell Bench Press: Warm-up and 3 hard sets	×	×	×
Seated Dumbbell Press: 3 hard sets	×	×	×
Dumbbell Side Lateral Raise: 3 hard sets	×	×	×
Seated Triceps Press: 3 hard sets	×	×	×
Crunch: 3 hard sets			

NOTES:

WORKOUT 3: LOWER BODY AND PULL (LEGS AND BACK)

EXERCISES	SETS		
Barbell Squat: Warm-up and 3 hard sets	×	×	×
Barbell Deadlift: Warm-up and 3 hard sets	×	×	×
One-Arm Dumbbell Row: 3 hard sets	×	×	×
Lat Pulldown (Wide-Grip): 3 hard sets	×	×	×
Barbell Curl: 3 hard sets	×	×	×

NOTES:

3-DAY ROUTINE	PHASE 1	WEEK 7

WORKOUT 1: LOWER BODY (LEGS AND GLUTES)

EXERCISES	SETS		
Barbell Squat: Warm-up and 3 hard sets	×	×	×
Leg Press: 3 hard sets	×	×	×
Romanian Deadlift: 3 hard sets	×	×	×
Hip Thrust: 3 hard sets	×	×	×

NOTES:

WORKOUT 2: UPPER BODY AND CORE

EXERCISES	SETS		
Barbell Bench Press: Warm-up and 3 hard sets	×	×	×
Seated Dumbbell Press: 3 hard sets	×	×	×
Dumbbell Side Lateral Raise: 3 hard sets	×	×	×
Seated Triceps Press: 3 hard sets	×	×	×
Crunch: 3 hard sets			

NOTES:

WORKOUT 3: LOWER BODY AND PULL (LEGS AND BACK)

EXERCISES	SETS		
Barbell Squat: Warm-up and 3 hard sets	×	×	×
Barbell Deadlift: Warm-up and 3 hard sets	×	×	×
One-Arm Dumbbell Row: 3 hard sets	×	×	×
Lat Pulldown (Wide-Grip): 3 hard sets	×	×	×
Barbell Curl: 3 hard sets	×	×	×

NOTES:

3-DAY ROUTINE	PHASE 1	WEEK 8

WORKOUT 1: LOWER BODY (LEGS AND GLUTES)

EXERCISES	SETS		
Barbell Squat: Warm-up and 3 hard sets	×	×	×
Leg Press: 3 hard sets	×	×	×
Romanian Deadlift: 3 hard sets	×	×	×
Hip Thrust: 3 hard sets	×	×	×

NOTES:

WORKOUT 2: UPPER BODY AND CORE

EXERCISES	SETS		
Barbell Bench Press: Warm-up and 3 hard sets	×	×	×
Seated Dumbbell Press: 3 hard sets	×	×	×
Dumbbell Side Lateral Raise: 3 hard sets	×	×	×
Seated Triceps Press: 3 hard sets	×	×	×
Crunch: 3 hard sets			

NOTES:

WORKOUT 3: LOWER BODY AND PULL (LEGS AND BACK)

EXERCISES	SETS		
Barbell Squat: Warm-up and 3 hard sets	×	×	×
Barbell Deadlift: Warm-up and 3 hard sets	×	×	×
One-Arm Dumbbell Row: 3 hard sets	×	×	×
Lat Pulldown (Wide-Grip): 3 hard sets	×	×	×
Barbell Curl: 3 hard sets	×	×	×

NOTES:

| 3-DAY ROUTINE | DELOAD | WEEK 9 |

WORKOUT 1: DELOAD LEGS

EXERCISES	SETS		
Barbell Squat: Warm-up and 3 sets of 5 reps with last hard set weight	×	×	×
Romanian Deadlift: 3 sets of 5 reps with last hard set weight	×	×	×
Hip Thrust: 3 sets of 5 reps with last hard set weight	×	×	×

NOTES:
_____
_____

WORKOUT 2: DELOAD PUSH

EXERCISES	SETS		
Barbell Bench Press: Warm-up and 3 sets of 5 reps with last hard set weight	×	×	×
Seated Dumbbell Press: 3 sets of 5 reps with last hard set weight	×	×	×
Dumbbell Bench Press: 3 sets of 5 reps with last hard set weight	×	×	×

NOTES:
_____
_____

WORKOUT 3: DELOAD PULL

EXERCISES	SETS		
Barbell Deadlift: Warm-up and 3 sets of 5 reps with last hard set weight	×	×	×
Barbell Row: 3 sets of 5 reps with last hard set weight	×	×	×
Lat Pulldown (Wide-Grip): 3 sets of 5 reps with last hard set weight	×	×	×

NOTES:
_____
_____

Great job on completing Phase 1!

You've been working hard for nine weeks, and by now, you should be totally comfortable with the exercises and with the weights that you can handle.

You should also notice changes in the mirror and how your clothes fit and most likely have gained or lost two to four pounds (depending on how you've set up your diet).

If you're excited about your progress and want to skip the deload/rest week and keep going, I totally understand—but don't do it!

Trust me—it's important to give your body a break every couple of months so it can get ready for the next block of training.

Which should you choose, though: deload, or rest?

I recommend that you start with a deload because most people find they don't need that much rest to recover from their first eight weeks of training. Later on, when you're a more advanced weightlifter lifting heavier weights, it can make more sense to take the occasional week off instead of deloading.

That said, if you're feeling worn down, then go ahead and take the week off. And if you want to get the absolute most out of the rest week, use the time you'd normally spend in the gym to get some extra sleep, as this works wonders for recovery.

Either that or use to the time for other interesting activities. Not only will this help you balance your social life with your newfound hobby, it also keeps you from getting bored, brooding about food, or fretting about your body.

Also, as far as your diet goes, you don't have to make any changes regardless of whether you're deloading to resting. If you're cutting, you'll just lose a little less fat this week (but alleviate some of the stress on your body), and if you're maintaining or lean bulking, the differences in long-term fat gain will be negligible.

You may find it more enjoyable to reduce your daily calories by about 10 percent if you're lean bulking though, simply to take a break from eating so much food. If that's the case, feel free to do so.

The last bit of housekeeping that we need to take care of before moving on is a new round of body measurements and progress pictures.

First, take the following body measurements first thing in the morning, nude, after using the bathroom and before eating or drinking anything:

1. Weight
2. Waist circumference
3. OPTIONAL: Hip circumference
4. OPTIONAL: Upper-leg circumference
5. OPTIONAL: Flexed arms

Then, take flexed and unflexed pictures from the front, back, and sides, and store them in an album or folder that you can easily locate.

Remember to show as much skin as you feel comfortable with. The more the better because it will give you the best idea of how your body is responding to the program.

All right, that's it for now!

Once you've finished the deload or rest week, you're ready to start Phase 2!

SOMETIMES DEATH ONLY COMES FROM A LACK OF ENERGY.

—NAPOLEON BONAPARTE

THINNER LEANER STRONGER PHASE 2

Congratulations on completing Phase 1, and welcome to Phase 2!

By now, you are comfortable with the key exercises of the program and acquainted with the weights you can handle, and you're seeing clear improvements in how your clothes fit and how you look in the mirror.

Fun, right?

Before you start Phase 2, please do make sure you've taken your deload or rest week. I know it's kind of boring and can feel like a waste of time, but it's important because it helps ensure you don't run into any symptoms related to overtraining. (I've been there and trust me, it's very annoying, not to mention unhealthy.)

On the following pages, you'll find your next eight weeks of hard training followed by a deload week. As before, choose the split that best suits your goals and circumstances, and stick with it until you've completed this second phase.

Before you start the first workout, let's do a quick exercise to help you get even more out of this second phase than the first.

Take a few minutes to reflect on the following questions, and if you have a lot to say, jot it down so you can easily refer back to it.

→ What are three things in your diet and/or training that went particularly well in the last phase? Why?

→ What's one thing you could have done better? Why?

→ What's one thing you can do to make your next phase even better than the last?

Okay, let's get to it!
Keep up the good work and see you soon!

5-DAY ROUTINE	PHASE 2	WEEK 10

WORKOUT 1: LOWER BODY (LEGS AND GLUTES)			
EXERCISES	**SETS**		
Barbell Squat: Warm-up and 3 hard sets	×	×	×
Dumbbell Lunge (In-Place): 3 hard sets	×	×	×
Leg Curl (Lying or Seated)*: 3 hard sets	×	×	×
Dumbbell Step-Up: 3 hard sets	×	×	×

NOTES:

WORKOUT 2: PUSH AND CORE			
EXERCISES	**SETS**		
Barbell Bench Press: Warm-up and 3 hard sets	×	×	×
Arnold Dumbbell Press: 3 hard sets	×	×	×
Dumbbell Bench Press: 3 hard sets	×	×	×
Barbell Rear Delt Row: 3 hard sets	×	×	×
Captain's Chair Leg Raise: 3 hard sets			

NOTES:

WORKOUT 3: PULL			
EXERCISES	**SETS**		
Barbell Deadlift: Warm-up and 3 hard sets	×	×	×
Barbell Row: 3 hard sets	×	×	×
Seated Cable Row (Wide-Grip): 3 hard sets	×	×	×
Dumbbell Hammer Curl: 3 hard sets	×	×	×

NOTES:

WORKOUT 4: UPPER BODY AND CORE			
EXERCISES	**SETS**		
Arnold Dumbbell Press: Warm-up and 3 hard sets	×	×	×
Close-Grip Bench Press: 3 hard sets	×	×	×
Dumbbell Side Lateral Raise: 3 hard sets	×	×	×
Lying Triceps Extension: 3 hard sets	×	×	×
Plank: 3 hard sets			

NOTES:

WORKOUT 5: LOWER BODY (LEGS AND GLUTES)			
EXERCISES	**SETS**		
Barbell Front Squat: Warm-up and 3 hard sets	×	×	×
Dumbbell Single-Leg Split Squat: 3 hard sets	×	×	×
Romanian Deadlift: 3 hard sets	×	×	×
Hip Thrust: 3 hard sets	×	×	×

NOTES:

5-DAY ROUTINE	PHASE 2	WEEK 11

WORKOUT 1: LOWER BODY (LEGS AND GLUTES)			
EXERCISES	**SETS**		
Barbell Squat: Warm-up and 3 hard sets	×	×	×
Dumbbell Lunge (In-Place): 3 hard sets	×	×	×
Leg Curl (Lying or Seated)*: 3 hard sets	×	×	×
Dumbbell Step-Up: 3 hard sets	×	×	×

NOTES:

WORKOUT 2: PUSH AND CORE			
EXERCISES	**SETS**		
Barbell Bench Press: Warm-up and 3 hard sets	×	×	×
Arnold Dumbbell Press: 3 hard sets	×	×	×
Dumbbell Bench Press: 3 hard sets	×	×	×
Barbell Rear Delt Row: 3 hard sets	×	×	×
Captain's Chair Leg Raise: 3 hard sets			

NOTES:

WORKOUT 3: PULL			
EXERCISES	**SETS**		
Barbell Deadlift: Warm-up and 3 hard sets	×	×	×
Barbell Row: 3 hard sets	×	×	×
Seated Cable Row (Wide-Grip): 3 hard sets	×	×	×
Dumbbell Hammer Curl: 3 hard sets	×	×	×

NOTES:

THE YEAR ONE CHALLENGE FOR WOMEN **135**

WORKOUT 4: UPPER BODY AND CORE			
EXERCISES	**SETS**		
Arnold Dumbbell Press: Warm-up and 3 hard sets	×	×	×
Close-Grip Bench Press: 3 hard sets	×	×	×
Dumbbell Side Lateral Raise: 3 hard sets	×	×	×
Lying Triceps Extension: 3 hard sets	×	×	×
Plank: 3 hard sets			

NOTES:

_____

_____

_____

WORKOUT 5: LOWER BODY (LEGS AND GLUTES)			
EXERCISES	**SETS**		
Barbell Front Squat: Warm-up and 3 hard sets	×	×	×
Dumbbell Single-Leg Split Squat: 3 hard sets	×	×	×
Romanian Deadlift: 3 hard sets	×	×	×
Hip Thrust: 3 hard sets	×	×	×

NOTES:

_____

_____

_____

5-DAY ROUTINE	PHASE 2	WEEK 12

WORKOUT 1: LOWER BODY (LEGS AND GLUTES)

EXERCISES	SETS		
Barbell Squat: Warm-up and 3 hard sets	×	×	×
Dumbbell Lunge (In-Place): 3 hard sets	×	×	×
Leg Curl (Lying or Seated)*: 3 hard sets	×	×	×
Dumbbell Step-Up: 3 hard sets	×	×	×

NOTES:

_____

_____

_____

WORKOUT 2: PUSH AND CORE

EXERCISES	SETS		
Barbell Bench Press: Warm-up and 3 hard sets	×	×	×
Arnold Dumbbell Press: 3 hard sets	×	×	×
Dumbbell Bench Press: 3 hard sets	×	×	×
Barbell Rear Delt Row: 3 hard sets	×	×	×
Captain's Chair Leg Raise: 3 hard sets			

NOTES:

_____

_____

_____

WORKOUT 3: PULL

EXERCISES	SETS		
Barbell Deadlift: Warm-up and 3 hard sets	×	×	×
Barbell Row: 3 hard sets	×	×	×
Seated Cable Row (Wide-Grip): 3 hard sets	×	×	×
Dumbbell Hammer Curl: 3 hard sets	×	×	×

NOTES:

_____

_____

_____

WORKOUT 4: UPPER BODY AND CORE			
EXERCISES	**SETS**		
Arnold Dumbbell Press: Warm-up and 3 hard sets	×	×	×
Close-Grip Bench Press: 3 hard sets	×	×	×
Dumbbell Side Lateral Raise: 3 hard sets	×	×	×
Lying Triceps Extension: 3 hard sets	×	×	×
Plank: 3 hard sets			

NOTES:

WORKOUT 5: LOWER BODY (LEGS AND GLUTES)			
EXERCISES	**SETS**		
Barbell Front Squat: Warm-up and 3 hard sets	×	×	×
Dumbbell Single-Leg Split Squat: 3 hard sets	×	×	×
Romanian Deadlift: 3 hard sets	×	×	×
Hip Thrust: 3 hard sets	×	×	×

NOTES:

5-DAY ROUTINE	PHASE 2	WEEK 13

WORKOUT 1: LOWER BODY (LEGS AND GLUTES)			
EXERCISES	**SETS**		
Barbell Squat: Warm-up and 3 hard sets	×	×	×
Dumbbell Lunge (In-Place): 3 hard sets	×	×	×
Leg Curl (Lying or Seated)*: 3 hard sets	×	×	×
Dumbbell Step-Up: 3 hard sets	×	×	×

NOTES:

WORKOUT 2: PUSH AND CORE			
EXERCISES	**SETS**		
Barbell Bench Press: Warm-up and 3 hard sets	×	×	×
Arnold Dumbbell Press: 3 hard sets	×	×	×
Dumbbell Bench Press: 3 hard sets	×	×	×
Barbell Rear Delt Row: 3 hard sets	×	×	×
Captain's Chair Leg Raise: 3 hard sets			

NOTES:

WORKOUT 3: PULL			
EXERCISES	**SETS**		
Barbell Deadlift: Warm-up and 3 hard sets	×	×	×
Barbell Row: 3 hard sets	×	×	×
Seated Cable Row (Wide-Grip): 3 hard sets	×	×	×
Dumbbell Hammer Curl: 3 hard sets	×	×	×

NOTES:

WORKOUT 4: UPPER BODY AND CORE			
EXERCISES	**SETS**		
Arnold Dumbbell Press: Warm-up and 3 hard sets	×	×	×
Close-Grip Bench Press: 3 hard sets	×	×	×
Dumbbell Side Lateral Raise: 3 hard sets	×	×	×
Lying Triceps Extension: 3 hard sets	×	×	×
Plank: 3 hard sets			

NOTES:

WORKOUT 5: LOWER BODY (LEGS AND GLUTES)			
EXERCISES	**SETS**		
Barbell Front Squat: Warm-up and 3 hard sets	×	×	×
Dumbbell Single-Leg Split Squat: 3 hard sets	×	×	×
Romanian Deadlift: 3 hard sets	×	×	×
Hip Thrust: 3 hard sets	×	×	×

NOTES:

5-DAY ROUTINE	PHASE 2	WEEK 14

WORKOUT 1: LOWER BODY (LEGS AND GLUTES)			
EXERCISES	SETS		
Barbell Squat: Warm-up and 3 hard sets	×	×	×
Dumbbell Lunge (In-Place): 3 hard sets	×	×	×
Leg Curl (Lying or Seated)*: 3 hard sets	×	×	×
Dumbbell Step-Up: 3 hard sets	×	×	×

NOTES:

WORKOUT 2: PUSH AND CORE			
EXERCISES	SETS		
Barbell Bench Press: Warm-up and 3 hard sets	×	×	×
Arnold Dumbbell Press: 3 hard sets	×	×	×
Dumbbell Bench Press: 3 hard sets	×	×	×
Barbell Rear Delt Row: 3 hard sets	×	×	×
Captain's Chair Leg Raise: 3 hard sets			

NOTES:

WORKOUT 3: PULL			
EXERCISES	SETS		
Barbell Deadlift: Warm-up and 3 hard sets	×	×	×
Barbell Row: 3 hard sets	×	×	×
Seated Cable Row (Wide-Grip): 3 hard sets	×	×	×
Dumbbell Hammer Curl: 3 hard sets	×	×	×

NOTES:

WORKOUT 4: UPPER BODY AND CORE			
EXERCISES	**SETS**		
Arnold Dumbbell Press: Warm-up and 3 hard sets	×	×	×
Close-Grip Bench Press: 3 hard sets	×	×	×
Dumbbell Side Lateral Raise: 3 hard sets	×	×	×
Lying Triceps Extension: 3 hard sets	×	×	×
Plank: 3 hard sets			

NOTES:

_____

_____

_____

WORKOUT 5: LOWER BODY (LEGS AND GLUTES)			
EXERCISES	**SETS**		
Barbell Front Squat: Warm-up and 3 hard sets	×	×	×
Dumbbell Single-Leg Split Squat: 3 hard sets	×	×	×
Romanian Deadlift: 3 hard sets	×	×	×
Hip Thrust: 3 hard sets	×	×	×

NOTES:

_____

_____

_____

5-DAY ROUTINE	PHASE 2	WEEK 15

WORKOUT 1: LOWER BODY (LEGS AND GLUTES)			
EXERCISES	SETS		
Barbell Squat: Warm-up and 3 hard sets	×	×	×
Dumbbell Lunge (In-Place): 3 hard sets	×	×	×
Leg Curl (Lying or Seated)*: 3 hard sets	×	×	×
Dumbbell Step-Up: 3 hard sets	×	×	×

NOTES:

WORKOUT 2: PUSH AND CORE			
EXERCISES	SETS		
Barbell Bench Press: Warm-up and 3 hard sets	×	×	×
Arnold Dumbbell Press: 3 hard sets	×	×	×
Dumbbell Bench Press: 3 hard sets	×	×	×
Barbell Rear Delt Row: 3 hard sets	×	×	×
Captain's Chair Leg Raise: 3 hard sets			

NOTES:

WORKOUT 3: PULL			
EXERCISES	SETS		
Barbell Deadlift: Warm-up and 3 hard sets	×	×	×
Barbell Row: 3 hard sets	×	×	×
Seated Cable Row (Wide-Grip): 3 hard sets	×	×	×
Dumbbell Hammer Curl: 3 hard sets	×	×	×

NOTES:

WORKOUT 4: UPPER BODY AND CORE			
EXERCISES	SETS		
Arnold Dumbbell Press: Warm-up and 3 hard sets	×	×	×
Close-Grip Bench Press: 3 hard sets	×	×	×
Dumbbell Side Lateral Raise: 3 hard sets	×	×	×
Lying Triceps Extension: 3 hard sets	×	×	×
Plank: 3 hard sets			

NOTES:

WORKOUT 5: LOWER BODY (LEGS AND GLUTES)			
EXERCISES	SETS		
Barbell Front Squat: Warm-up and 3 hard sets	×	×	×
Dumbbell Single-Leg Split Squat: 3 hard sets	×	×	×
Romanian Deadlift: 3 hard sets	×	×	×
Hip Thrust: 3 hard sets	×	×	×

NOTES:

| 5-DAY ROUTINE | PHASE 2 | WEEK 16 |

WORKOUT 1: LOWER BODY (LEGS AND GLUTES)			
EXERCISES	SETS		
Barbell Squat: Warm-up and 3 hard sets	×	×	×
Dumbbell Lunge (In-Place): 3 hard sets	×	×	×
Leg Curl (Lying or Seated)*: 3 hard sets	×	×	×
Dumbbell Step-Up: 3 hard sets	×	×	×

NOTES:

WORKOUT 2: PUSH AND CORE			
EXERCISES	SETS		
Barbell Bench Press: Warm-up and 3 hard sets	×	×	×
Arnold Dumbbell Press: 3 hard sets	×	×	×
Dumbbell Bench Press: 3 hard sets	×	×	×
Barbell Rear Delt Row: 3 hard sets	×	×	×
Captain's Chair Leg Raise: 3 hard sets			

NOTES:

WORKOUT 3: PULL			
EXERCISES	SETS		
Barbell Deadlift: Warm-up and 3 hard sets	×	×	×
Barbell Row: 3 hard sets	×	×	×
Seated Cable Row (Wide-Grip): 3 hard sets	×	×	×
Dumbbell Hammer Curl: 3 hard sets	×	×	×

NOTES:

WORKOUT 4: UPPER BODY AND CORE			
EXERCISES	**SETS**		
Arnold Dumbbell Press: Warm-up and 3 hard sets	×	×	×
Close-Grip Bench Press: 3 hard sets	×	×	×
Dumbbell Side Lateral Raise: 3 hard sets	×	×	×
Lying Triceps Extension: 3 hard sets	×	×	×
Plank: 3 hard sets			

NOTES:

WORKOUT 5: LOWER BODY (LEGS AND GLUTES)			
EXERCISES	**SETS**		
Barbell Front Squat: Warm-up and 3 hard sets	×	×	×
Dumbbell Single-Leg Split Squat: 3 hard sets	×	×	×
Romanian Deadlift: 3 hard sets	×	×	×
Hip Thrust: 3 hard sets	×	×	×

NOTES:

5-DAY ROUTINE	PHASE 2	WEEK 17

WORKOUT 1: LOWER BODY (LEGS AND GLUTES)			
EXERCISES	SETS		
Barbell Squat: Warm-up and 3 hard sets	×	×	×
Dumbbell Lunge (In-Place): 3 hard sets	×	×	×
Leg Curl (Lying or Seated)*: 3 hard sets	×	×	×
Dumbbell Step-Up: 3 hard sets	×	×	×

NOTES:

WORKOUT 2: PUSH AND CORE			
EXERCISES	SETS		
Barbell Bench Press: Warm-up and 3 hard sets	×	×	×
Arnold Dumbbell Press: 3 hard sets	×	×	×
Dumbbell Bench Press: 3 hard sets	×	×	×
Barbell Rear Delt Row: 3 hard sets	×	×	×
Captain's Chair Leg Raise: 3 hard sets			

NOTES:

WORKOUT 3: PULL			
EXERCISES	SETS		
Barbell Deadlift: Warm-up and 3 hard sets	×	×	×
Barbell Row: 3 hard sets	×	×	×
Seated Cable Row (Wide-Grip): 3 hard sets	×	×	×
Dumbbell Hammer Curl: 3 hard sets	×	×	×

NOTES:

WORKOUT 4: UPPER BODY AND CORE			
EXERCISES	**SETS**		
Arnold Dumbbell Press: Warm-up and 3 hard sets	×	×	×
Close-Grip Bench Press: 3 hard sets	×	×	×
Dumbbell Side Lateral Raise: 3 hard sets	×	×	×
Lying Triceps Extension: 3 hard sets	×	×	×
Plank: 3 hard sets			

NOTES:

_____

_____

_____

WORKOUT 5: LOWER BODY (LEGS AND GLUTES)			
EXERCISES	**SETS**		
Barbell Front Squat: Warm-up and 3 hard sets	×	×	×
Dumbbell Single-Leg Split Squat: 3 hard sets	×	×	×
Romanian Deadlift: 3 hard sets	×	×	×
Hip Thrust: 3 hard sets	×	×	×

NOTES:

_____

_____

_____

5-DAY ROUTINE	DELOAD	WEEK 18

WORKOUT 1: DELOAD LEGS

EXERCISES	SETS		
Barbell Squat: Warm-up and 3 sets of 5 reps with last hard set weight	×	×	×
Romanian Deadlift: 3 sets of 5 reps with last hard set weight	×	×	×
Hip Thrust: 3 sets of 5 reps with last hard set weight	×	×	×

NOTES:

WORKOUT 2: DELOAD PUSH

EXERCISES	SETS		
Barbell Bench Press: Warm-up and 3 sets of 5 reps with last hard set weight	×	×	×
Seated Dumbbell Press: 3 sets of 5 reps with last hard set weight	×	×	×
Dumbbell Side Lateral Raise: 3 sets of 5 reps with last hard set weight	×	×	×

NOTES:

WORKOUT 3: DELOAD PULL

EXERCISES	SETS		
Barbell Deadlift: Warm-up and 3 sets of 5 reps with last hard set weight	×	×	×
Barbell Row: 3 sets of 5 reps with last hard set weight	×	×	×
Lat Pulldown (Wide-Grip): 3 sets of 5 reps with last hard set weight	×	×	×

NOTES:

4-DAY ROUTINE	PHASE 2	WEEK 10

WORKOUT 1: LOWER BODY (LEGS AND GLUTES)

EXERCISES	SETS		
Barbell Squat: Warm-up and 3 hard sets	×	×	×
Dumbbell Lunge (In-Place): 3 hard sets	×	×	×
Leg Curl (Lying or Seated)*: 3 hard sets	×	×	×
Dumbbell Step-Up: 3 hard sets	×	×	×

NOTES:
_____
_____
_____

WORKOUT 2: UPPER BODY AND CORE

EXERCISES	SETS		
Barbell Bench Press: Warm-up and 3 hard sets	×	×	×
Arnold Dumbbell Press: 3 hard sets	×	×	×
Barbell Rear Delt Row: 3 hard sets	×	×	×
Lying Triceps Extension: 3 hard sets	×	×	×
Plank: 3 hard sets			

NOTES:
_____
_____
_____

WORKOUT 3: PULL			
EXERCISES	**SETS**		
Barbell Deadlift: Warm-up and 3 hard sets	✕	✕	✕
Barbell Row: 3 hard sets	✕	✕	✕
Seated Cable Row (Wide-Grip): 3 hard sets	✕	✕	✕
Dumbbell Hammer Curl: 3 hard sets	✕	✕	✕

NOTES:

_____

_____

_____

WORKOUT 4: LOWER BODY (LEGS AND GLUTES)			
EXERCISES	**SETS**		
Barbell Squat: Warm-up and 3 hard sets	✕	✕	✕
Dumbbell Single-Leg Split Squat: 3 hard sets	✕	✕	✕
Romanian Deadlift: 3 hard sets	✕	✕	✕
Hip Thrust: 3 hard sets	✕	✕	✕

NOTES:

_____

_____

_____

4-DAY ROUTINE	PHASE 2	WEEK 11

WORKOUT 1: LOWER BODY (LEGS AND GLUTES)

EXERCISES	SETS		
Barbell Squat: Warm-up and 3 hard sets	×	×	×
Dumbbell Lunge (In-Place): 3 hard sets	×	×	×
Leg Curl (Lying or Seated)*: 3 hard sets	×	×	×
Dumbbell Step-Up: 3 hard sets	×	×	×

NOTES:

_____

_____

_____

WORKOUT 2: UPPER BODY AND CORE

EXERCISES	SETS		
Barbell Bench Press: Warm-up and 3 hard sets	×	×	×
Arnold Dumbbell Press: 3 hard sets	×	×	×
Barbell Rear Delt Row: 3 hard sets	×	×	×
Lying Triceps Extension: 3 hard sets	×	×	×
Plank: 3 hard sets			

NOTES:

_____

_____

_____

WORKOUT 3: PULL			
EXERCISES	**SETS**		
Barbell Deadlift: Warm-up and 3 hard sets	✕	✕	✕
Barbell Row: 3 hard sets	✕	✕	✕
Seated Cable Row (Wide-Grip): 3 hard sets	✕	✕	✕
Dumbbell Hammer Curl: 3 hard sets	✕	✕	✕

NOTES:
_____
_____
_____

WORKOUT 4: LOWER BODY (LEGS AND GLUTES)			
EXERCISES	**SETS**		
Barbell Squat: Warm-up and 3 hard sets	✕	✕	✕
Dumbbell Single-Leg Split Squat: 3 hard sets	✕	✕	✕
Romanian Deadlift: 3 hard sets	✕	✕	✕
Hip Thrust: 3 hard sets	✕	✕	✕

NOTES:
_____
_____
_____

4-DAY ROUTINE	PHASE 2	WEEK 12

WORKOUT 1: LOWER BODY (LEGS AND GLUTES)

EXERCISES	SETS		
Barbell Squat: Warm-up and 3 hard sets	×	×	×
Dumbbell Lunge (In-Place): 3 hard sets	×	×	×
Leg Curl (Lying or Seated)*: 3 hard sets	×	×	×
Dumbbell Step-Up: 3 hard sets	×	×	×

NOTES:

WORKOUT 2: UPPER BODY AND CORE

EXERCISES	SETS		
Barbell Bench Press: Warm-up and 3 hard sets	×	×	×
Arnold Dumbbell Press: 3 hard sets	×	×	×
Barbell Rear Delt Row: 3 hard sets	×	×	×
Lying Triceps Extension: 3 hard sets	×	×	×
Plank: 3 hard sets			

NOTES:

WORKOUT 3: PULL			
EXERCISES	**SETS**		
Barbell Deadlift: Warm-up and 3 hard sets	×	×	×
Barbell Row: 3 hard sets	×	×	×
Seated Cable Row (Wide-Grip): 3 hard sets	×	×	×
Dumbbell Hammer Curl: 3 hard sets	×	×	×

NOTES:

WORKOUT 4: LOWER BODY (LEGS AND GLUTES)			
EXERCISES	**SETS**		
Barbell Squat: Warm-up and 3 hard sets	×	×	×
Dumbbell Single-Leg Split Squat: 3 hard sets	×	×	×
Romanian Deadlift: 3 hard sets	×	×	×
Hip Thrust: 3 hard sets	×	×	×

NOTES:

4-DAY ROUTINE	PHASE 2	WEEK 13

WORKOUT 1: LOWER BODY (LEGS AND GLUTES)

EXERCISES	SETS		
Barbell Squat: Warm-up and 3 hard sets	×	×	×
Dumbbell Lunge (In-Place): 3 hard sets	×	×	×
Leg Curl (Lying or Seated)*: 3 hard sets	×	×	×
Dumbbell Step-Up: 3 hard sets	×	×	×

NOTES:

WORKOUT 2: UPPER BODY AND CORE

EXERCISES	SETS		
Barbell Bench Press: Warm-up and 3 hard sets	×	×	×
Arnold Dumbbell Press: 3 hard sets	×	×	×
Barbell Rear Delt Row: 3 hard sets	×	×	×
Lying Triceps Extension: 3 hard sets	×	×	×
Plank: 3 hard sets			

NOTES:

WORKOUT 3: PULL			
EXERCISES	**SETS**		
Barbell Deadlift: Warm-up and 3 hard sets	×	×	×
Barbell Row: 3 hard sets	×	×	×
Seated Cable Row (Wide-Grip): 3 hard sets	×	×	×
Dumbbell Hammer Curl: 3 hard sets	×	×	×

NOTES:

_____

_____

_____

WORKOUT 4: LOWER BODY (LEGS AND GLUTES)			
EXERCISES	**SETS**		
Barbell Squat: Warm-up and 3 hard sets	×	×	×
Dumbbell Single-Leg Split Squat: 3 hard sets	×	×	×
Romanian Deadlift: 3 hard sets	×	×	×
Hip Thrust: 3 hard sets	×	×	×

NOTES:

_____

_____

_____

4-DAY ROUTINE	PHASE 2	WEEK 14

WORKOUT 1: LOWER BODY (LEGS AND GLUTES)

EXERCISES	SETS		
Barbell Squat: Warm-up and 3 hard sets	×	×	×
Dumbbell Lunge (In-Place): 3 hard sets	×	×	×
Leg Curl (Lying or Seated)*: 3 hard sets	×	×	×
Dumbbell Step-Up: 3 hard sets	×	×	×

NOTES:

WORKOUT 2: UPPER BODY AND CORE

EXERCISES	SETS		
Barbell Bench Press: Warm-up and 3 hard sets	×	×	×
Arnold Dumbbell Press: 3 hard sets	×	×	×
Barbell Rear Delt Row: 3 hard sets	×	×	×
Lying Triceps Extension: 3 hard sets	×	×	×
Plank: 3 hard sets			

NOTES:

WORKOUT 3: PULL			
EXERCISES	**SETS**		
Barbell Deadlift: Warm-up and 3 hard sets	×	×	×
Barbell Row: 3 hard sets	×	×	×
Seated Cable Row (Wide-Grip): 3 hard sets	×	×	×
Dumbbell Hammer Curl: 3 hard sets	×	×	×

NOTES:

WORKOUT 4: LOWER BODY (LEGS AND GLUTES)			
EXERCISES	**SETS**		
Barbell Squat: Warm-up and 3 hard sets	×	×	×
Dumbbell Single-Leg Split Squat: 3 hard sets	×	×	×
Romanian Deadlift: 3 hard sets	×	×	×
Hip Thrust: 3 hard sets	×	×	×

NOTES:

| 4-DAY ROUTINE | PHASE 2 | WEEK 15 |

WORKOUT 1: LOWER BODY (LEGS AND GLUTES)

EXERCISES	SETS		
Barbell Squat: Warm-up and 3 hard sets	×	×	×
Dumbbell Lunge (In-Place): 3 hard sets	×	×	×
Leg Curl (Lying or Seated)*: 3 hard sets	×	×	×
Dumbbell Step-Up: 3 hard sets	×	×	×

NOTES:

WORKOUT 2: UPPER BODY AND CORE

EXERCISES	SETS		
Barbell Bench Press: Warm-up and 3 hard sets	×	×	×
Arnold Dumbbell Press: 3 hard sets	×	×	×
Barbell Rear Delt Row: 3 hard sets	×	×	×
Lying Triceps Extension: 3 hard sets	×	×	×
Plank: 3 hard sets			

NOTES:

WORKOUT 3: PULL			
EXERCISES	**SETS**		
Barbell Deadlift: Warm-up and 3 hard sets	×	×	×
Barbell Row: 3 hard sets	×	×	×
Seated Cable Row (Wide-Grip): 3 hard sets	×	×	×
Dumbbell Hammer Curl: 3 hard sets	×	×	×

NOTES:

_____

_____

WORKOUT 4: LOWER BODY (LEGS AND GLUTES)			
EXERCISES	**SETS**		
Barbell Squat: Warm-up and 3 hard sets	×	×	×
Dumbbell Single-Leg Split Squat: 3 hard sets	×	×	×
Romanian Deadlift: 3 hard sets	×	×	×
Hip Thrust: 3 hard sets	×	×	×

NOTES:

_____

_____

| 4-DAY ROUTINE | PHASE 2 | WEEK 16 |

WORKOUT 1: LOWER BODY (LEGS AND GLUTES)

EXERCISES	SETS		
Barbell Squat: Warm-up and 3 hard sets	×	×	×
Dumbbell Lunge (In-Place): 3 hard sets	×	×	×
Leg Curl (Lying or Seated)*: 3 hard sets	×	×	×
Dumbbell Step-Up: 3 hard sets	×	×	×

NOTES:

WORKOUT 2: UPPER BODY AND CORE

EXERCISES	SETS		
Barbell Bench Press: Warm-up and 3 hard sets	×	×	×
Arnold Dumbbell Press: 3 hard sets	×	×	×
Barbell Rear Delt Row: 3 hard sets	×	×	×
Lying Triceps Extension: 3 hard sets	×	×	×
Plank: 3 hard sets			

NOTES:

WORKOUT 3: PULL			
EXERCISES	**SETS**		
Barbell Deadlift: Warm-up and 3 hard sets	×	×	×
Barbell Row: 3 hard sets	×	×	×
Seated Cable Row (Wide-Grip): 3 hard sets	×	×	×
Dumbbell Hammer Curl: 3 hard sets	×	×	×

NOTES:

WORKOUT 4: LOWER BODY (LEGS AND GLUTES)			
EXERCISES	**SETS**		
Barbell Squat: Warm-up and 3 hard sets	×	×	×
Dumbbell Single-Leg Split Squat: 3 hard sets	×	×	×
Romanian Deadlift: 3 hard sets	×	×	×
Hip Thrust: 3 hard sets	×	×	×

NOTES:

4-DAY ROUTINE	PHASE 2	WEEK 17

WORKOUT 1: LOWER BODY (LEGS AND GLUTES)			
EXERCISES	**SETS**		
Barbell Squat: Warm-up and 3 hard sets	×	×	×
Dumbbell Lunge (In-Place): 3 hard sets	×	×	×
Leg Curl (Lying or Seated)*: 3 hard sets	×	×	×
Dumbbell Step-Up: 3 hard sets	×	×	×

NOTES:
_____
_____
_____

WORKOUT 2: UPPER BODY AND CORE			
EXERCISES	**SETS**		
Barbell Bench Press: Warm-up and 3 hard sets	×	×	×
Arnold Dumbbell Press: 3 hard sets	×	×	×
Barbell Rear Delt Row: 3 hard sets	×	×	×
Lying Triceps Extension: 3 hard sets	×	×	×
Plank: 3 hard sets			

NOTES:
_____
_____
_____

WORKOUT 3: PULL			
EXERCISES	SETS		
Barbell Deadlift: Warm-up and 3 hard sets	×	×	×
Barbell Row: 3 hard sets	×	×	×
Seated Cable Row (Wide-Grip): 3 hard sets	×	×	×
Dumbbell Hammer Curl: 3 hard sets	×	×	×

NOTES:

_____

_____

_____

WORKOUT 4: LOWER BODY (LEGS AND GLUTES)			
EXERCISES	SETS		
Barbell Squat: Warm-up and 3 hard sets	×	×	×
Dumbbell Single-Leg Split Squat: 3 hard sets	×	×	×
Romanian Deadlift: 3 hard sets	×	×	×
Hip Thrust: 3 hard sets	×	×	×

NOTES:

_____

_____

_____

4-DAY ROUTINE | DELOAD | WEEK 18

WORKOUT 1: DELOAD LEGS

EXERCISES	SETS		
Barbell Squat: Warm-up and 3 sets of 5 reps with last hard set weight	×	×	×
Romanian Deadlift: 3 sets of 5 reps with last hard set weight	×	×	×
Hip Thrust: 3 sets of 5 reps with last hard set weight	×	×	×

NOTES:

WORKOUT 2: DELOAD PUSH

EXERCISES	SETS		
Barbell Bench Press: Warm-up and 3 sets of 5 reps with last hard set weight	×	×	×
Seated Dumbbell Press: 3 sets of 5 reps with last hard set weight	×	×	×
Dumbbell Bench Press: 3 sets of 5 reps with last hard set weight	×	×	×

NOTES:

WORKOUT 3: DELOAD PULL

EXERCISES	SETS		
Barbell Deadlift: Warm-up and 3 sets of 5 reps with last hard set weight	×	×	×
Barbell Row: 3 sets of 5 reps with last hard set weight	×	×	×
Lat Pulldown (Wide-Grip): 3 sets of 5 reps with last hard set weight	×	×	×

NOTES:

| 3-DAY ROUTINE | PHASE 2 | WEEK 10 |

WORKOUT 1: LOWER BODY (LEGS AND GLUTES)

EXERCISES	SETS		
Barbell Squat: Warm-up and 3 hard sets	×	×	×
Dumbbell Lunge (In-Place): 3 hard sets	×	×	×
Leg Curl (Lying or Seated)*: 3 hard sets	×	×	×
Dumbbell Step-Up: 3 hard sets	×	×	×

NOTES:

WORKOUT 2: UPPER BODY AND CORE

EXERCISES	SETS		
Barbell Bench Press: Warm-up and 3 hard sets	×	×	×
Arnold Dumbbell Press: 3 hard sets	×	×	×
Barbell Rear Delt Row: 3 hard sets	×	×	×
Lying Triceps Extension: 3 hard sets	×	×	×
Captain's Chair Leg Raise: 3 hard sets			

NOTES:

WORKOUT 3: LOWER BODY AND PULL (LEGS AND BACK)

EXERCISES	SETS		
Barbell Squat: Warm-up and 3 hard sets	×	×	×
Barbell Deadlift: Warm-up and 3 hard sets	×	×	×
Lat Pulldown (Close-Grip): 3 hard sets	×	×	×
Seated Cable Row (Wide-Grip): 3 hard sets	×	×	×
Dumbbell Hammer Curl: 3 hard sets	×	×	×

NOTES:

3-DAY ROUTINE | PHASE 2 | WEEK 11

WORKOUT 1: LOWER BODY (LEGS AND GLUTES)

EXERCISES	SETS		
Barbell Squat: Warm-up and 3 hard sets	×	×	×
Dumbbell Lunge (In-Place): 3 hard sets	×	×	×
Leg Curl (Lying or Seated)*: 3 hard sets	×	×	×
Dumbbell Step-Up: 3 hard sets	×	×	×

NOTES:

WORKOUT 2: UPPER BODY AND CORE

EXERCISES	SETS		
Barbell Bench Press: Warm-up and 3 hard sets	×	×	×
Arnold Dumbbell Press: 3 hard sets	×	×	×
Barbell Rear Delt Row: 3 hard sets	×	×	×
Lying Triceps Extension: 3 hard sets	×	×	×
Captain's Chair Leg Raise: 3 hard sets			

NOTES:

WORKOUT 3: LOWER BODY AND PULL (LEGS AND BACK)

EXERCISES	SETS		
Barbell Squat: Warm-up and 3 hard sets	×	×	×
Barbell Deadlift: Warm-up and 3 hard sets	×	×	×
Lat Pulldown (Close-Grip): 3 hard sets	×	×	×
Seated Cable Row (Wide-Grip): 3 hard sets	×	×	×
Dumbbell Hammer Curl: 3 hard sets	×	×	×

NOTES:

| 3-DAY ROUTINE | PHASE 2 | WEEK 12 |

WORKOUT 1: LOWER BODY (LEGS AND GLUTES)			
EXERCISES	SETS		
Barbell Squat: Warm-up and 3 hard sets	×	×	×
Dumbbell Lunge (In-Place): 3 hard sets	×	×	×
Leg Curl (Lying or Seated)*: 3 hard sets	×	×	×
Dumbbell Step-Up: 3 hard sets	×	×	×

NOTES:

WORKOUT 2: UPPER BODY AND CORE			
EXERCISES	SETS		
Barbell Bench Press: Warm-up and 3 hard sets	×	×	×
Arnold Dumbbell Press: 3 hard sets	×	×	×
Barbell Rear Delt Row: 3 hard sets	×	×	×
Lying Triceps Extension: 3 hard sets	×	×	×
Captain's Chair Leg Raise: 3 hard sets			

NOTES:

WORKOUT 3: LOWER BODY AND PULL (LEGS AND BACK)			
EXERCISES	SETS		
Barbell Squat: Warm-up and 3 hard sets	×	×	×
Barbell Deadlift: Warm-up and 3 hard sets	×	×	×
Lat Pulldown (Close-Grip): 3 hard sets	×	×	×
Seated Cable Row (Wide-Grip): 3 hard sets	×	×	×
Dumbbell Hammer Curl: 3 hard sets	×	×	×

NOTES:

3-DAY ROUTINE	PHASE 2	WEEK 13

WORKOUT 1: LOWER BODY (LEGS AND GLUTES)

EXERCISES	SETS		
Barbell Squat: Warm-up and 3 hard sets	×	×	×
Dumbbell Lunge (In-Place): 3 hard sets	×	×	×
Leg Curl (Lying or Seated)*: 3 hard sets	×	×	×
Dumbbell Step-Up: 3 hard sets	×	×	×

NOTES:

WORKOUT 2: UPPER BODY AND CORE

EXERCISES	SETS		
Barbell Bench Press: Warm-up and 3 hard sets	×	×	×
Arnold Dumbbell Press: 3 hard sets	×	×	×
Barbell Rear Delt Row: 3 hard sets	×	×	×
Lying Triceps Extension: 3 hard sets	×	×	×
Captain's Chair Leg Raise: 3 hard sets			

NOTES:

WORKOUT 3: LOWER BODY AND PULL (LEGS AND BACK)

EXERCISES	SETS		
Barbell Squat: Warm-up and 3 hard sets	×	×	×
Barbell Deadlift: Warm-up and 3 hard sets	×	×	×
Lat Pulldown (Close-Grip): 3 hard sets	×	×	×
Seated Cable Row (Wide-Grip): 3 hard sets	×	×	×
Dumbbell Hammer Curl: 3 hard sets	×	×	×

NOTES:

3-DAY ROUTINE	PHASE 2	WEEK 14

WORKOUT 1: LOWER BODY (LEGS AND GLUTES)

EXERCISES	SETS		
Barbell Squat: Warm-up and 3 hard sets	×	×	×
Dumbbell Lunge (In-Place): 3 hard sets	×	×	×
Leg Curl (Lying or Seated)*: 3 hard sets	×	×	×
Dumbbell Step-Up: 3 hard sets	×	×	×

NOTES:

WORKOUT 2: UPPER BODY AND CORE

EXERCISES	SETS		
Barbell Bench Press: Warm-up and 3 hard sets	×	×	×
Arnold Dumbbell Press: 3 hard sets	×	×	×
Barbell Rear Delt Row: 3 hard sets	×	×	×
Lying Triceps Extension: 3 hard sets	×	×	×
Captain's Chair Leg Raise: 3 hard sets			

NOTES:

WORKOUT 3: LOWER BODY AND PULL (LEGS AND BACK)

EXERCISES	SETS		
Barbell Squat: Warm-up and 3 hard sets	×	×	×
Barbell Deadlift: Warm-up and 3 hard sets	×	×	×
Lat Pulldown (Close-Grip): 3 hard sets	×	×	×
Seated Cable Row (Wide-Grip): 3 hard sets	×	×	×
Dumbbell Hammer Curl: 3 hard sets	×	×	×

NOTES:

| 3-DAY ROUTINE | PHASE 2 | WEEK 15 |

WORKOUT 1: LOWER BODY (LEGS AND GLUTES)

EXERCISES	SETS		
Barbell Squat: Warm-up and 3 hard sets	×	×	×
Dumbbell Lunge (In-Place): 3 hard sets	×	×	×
Leg Curl (Lying or Seated)*: 3 hard sets	×	×	×
Dumbbell Step-Up: 3 hard sets	×	×	×

NOTES:

WORKOUT 2: UPPER BODY AND CORE

EXERCISES	SETS		
Barbell Bench Press: Warm-up and 3 hard sets	×	×	×
Arnold Dumbbell Press: 3 hard sets	×	×	×
Barbell Rear Delt Row: 3 hard sets	×	×	×
Lying Triceps Extension: 3 hard sets	×	×	×
Captain's Chair Leg Raise: 3 hard sets			

NOTES:

WORKOUT 3: LOWER BODY AND PULL (LEGS AND BACK)

EXERCISES	SETS		
Barbell Squat: Warm-up and 3 hard sets	×	×	×
Barbell Deadlift: Warm-up and 3 hard sets	×	×	×
Lat Pulldown (Close-Grip): 3 hard sets	×	×	×
Seated Cable Row (Wide-Grip): 3 hard sets	×	×	×
Dumbbell Hammer Curl: 3 hard sets	×	×	×

NOTES:

3-DAY ROUTINE	PHASE 2	WEEK 16

WORKOUT 1: LOWER BODY (LEGS AND GLUTES)			
EXERCISES	**SETS**		
Barbell Squat: Warm-up and 3 hard sets	×	×	×
Dumbbell Lunge (In-Place): 3 hard sets	×	×	×
Leg Curl (Lying or Seated)*: 3 hard sets	×	×	×
Dumbbell Step-Up: 3 hard sets	×	×	×

NOTES:

WORKOUT 2: UPPER BODY AND CORE			
EXERCISES	**SETS**		
Barbell Bench Press: Warm-up and 3 hard sets	×	×	×
Arnold Dumbbell Press: 3 hard sets	×	×	×
Barbell Rear Delt Row: 3 hard sets	×	×	×
Lying Triceps Extension: 3 hard sets	×	×	×
Captain's Chair Leg Raise: 3 hard sets			

NOTES:

WORKOUT 3: LOWER BODY AND PULL (LEGS AND BACK)			
EXERCISES	**SETS**		
Barbell Squat: Warm-up and 3 hard sets	×	×	×
Barbell Deadlift: Warm-up and 3 hard sets	×	×	×
Lat Pulldown (Close-Grip): 3 hard sets	×	×	×
Seated Cable Row (Wide-Grip): 3 hard sets	×	×	×
Dumbbell Hammer Curl: 3 hard sets	×	×	×

NOTES:

3-DAY ROUTINE	PHASE 2	WEEK 17

WORKOUT 1: LOWER BODY (LEGS AND GLUTES)

EXERCISES	SETS		
Barbell Squat: Warm-up and 3 hard sets	×	×	×
Dumbbell Lunge (In-Place): 3 hard sets	×	×	×
Leg Curl (Lying or Seated)*: 3 hard sets	×	×	×
Dumbbell Step-Up: 3 hard sets	×	×	×

NOTES:

WORKOUT 2: UPPER BODY AND CORE

EXERCISES	SETS		
Barbell Bench Press: Warm-up and 3 hard sets	×	×	×
Arnold Dumbbell Press: 3 hard sets	×	×	×
Barbell Rear Delt Row: 3 hard sets	×	×	×
Lying Triceps Extension: 3 hard sets	×	×	×
Captain's Chair Leg Raise: 3 hard sets			

NOTES:

WORKOUT 3: LOWER BODY AND PULL (LEGS AND BACK)

EXERCISES	SETS		
Barbell Squat: Warm-up and 3 hard sets	×	×	×
Barbell Deadlift: Warm-up and 3 hard sets	×	×	×
Lat Pulldown (Close-Grip): 3 hard sets	×	×	×
Seated Cable Row (Wide-Grip): 3 hard sets	×	×	×
Dumbbell Hammer Curl: 3 hard sets	×	×	×

NOTES:

3-DAY ROUTINE | DELOAD | WEEK 18

WORKOUT 1: DELOAD LEGS

EXERCISES	SETS		
Barbell Squat: Warm-up and 3 sets of 5 reps with last hard set weight	×	×	×
Romanian Deadlift: 3 sets of 5 reps with last hard set weight	×	×	×
Hip Thrust: 3 sets of 5 reps with last hard set weight	×	×	×

NOTES:

WORKOUT 2: DELOAD PUSH

EXERCISES	SETS		
Barbell Bench Press: Warm-up and 3 sets of 5 reps with last hard set weight	×	×	×
Seated Dumbbell Press: 3 sets of 5 reps with last hard set weight	×	×	×
Dumbbell Bench Press: 3 sets of 5 reps with last hard set weight	×	×	×

NOTES:

WORKOUT 3: DELOAD PULL

EXERCISES	SETS		
Barbell Deadlift: Warm-up and 3 sets of 5 reps with last hard set weight	×	×	×
Barbell Row: 3 sets of 5 reps with last hard set weight	×	×	×
Lat Pulldown (Wide-Grip): 3 sets of 5 reps with last hard set weight	×	×	×

NOTES:

And just like that, Phase 2 is done! Good work!

That means new personal records (PRs), more inches shed (or gained if you're lean bulking!), and a sexier you staring back in the mirror every day.

This also calls for a special celebration. I want you to treat yourself to a nice reward. A cheat meal that you've been hankering for, maybe? :-)

And what exactly are we celebrating, you ask? The fact that you've made it past the third month—which for some odd reason is where so many people give up on their fitness journeys. You didn't though, which means you're awesome!

Also worth celebrating: the fact that by now, your daily training and eating regimens are probably starting to feel like an integral and essential part of your life, and people are probably starting to notice it.

If you haven't already, get ready to be asked, "Wow, are you working out?" by pretty much everyone you know. They'll probably start asking you for advice, too!

Before you rip into Phase 3, remember to take your deload or rest week to boost your recovery and prepare your body for the next couple of months, and to take a new round of measurements and pictures.

First, take the following body measurements first thing in the morning, nude, after using the bathroom and before eating or drinking anything:

1. Weight
2. Waist circumference
3. OPTIONAL: Hip circumference
4. OPTIONAL: Upper-leg circumference
5. OPTIONAL: Flexed arms

Then, take flexed and unflexed pictures from the front, back, and sides, and store them in an album or folder that you can easily locate later.

Remember to show as much skin as you feel comfortable with. The more the better because it will give you the best idea of how your body is responding to the program.

Carry on!

IF YOU HAVE EVERYTHING UNDER CONTROL, YOU'RE NOT MOVING FAST ENOUGH.

—MARIO ANDRETTI

THINNER LEANER STRONGER PHASE 3

Congratulations on completing Phase 2, and welcome to Phase 3!

I wouldn't go so far as to say "it's all downhill from here," but it's certainly easier to keep showing up now that you've firmly established the habit. If they aren't already, your new diet and exercise routines will become your new default—your new lifestyle. And that's the ultimate goal: long-term, sustainable fitness and health.

So, let's talk Phase 3.

On the following pages, you'll find your next nine weeks of *Thinner Leaner Stronger*. As before, choose the split that best suits your goals and circumstances, and stick with it until you've completed this third phase.

This phase is a bit tougher than the last, but I'm not going to ask you to do anything that you can't do.

You should be feeling fresh after your deload or rest week, so hit these next workouts with the same intensity and determination that has gotten you this far, and get ready to set some new PRs!

Just like we did last time, let's take a moment to reflect on how the last nine weeks went before forging ahead.

Reflect on the following questions, and if you have a lot to say, jot it down so you can easily refer back to it.

→ What are three things in your diet and/or training that went particularly well in the last phase? Why?

→ What's one thing you could have done better? Why?

→ What's one thing you can do to make your next phase even better than the last?

Done? Perfect. To the gym with thee! :-)

5-DAY ROUTINE	PHASE 3	WEEK 19

WORKOUT 1: LOWER BODY (LEGS AND GLUTES)			
EXERCISES	**SETS**		
Barbell Squat: Warm-up and 3 hard sets	×	×	×
Dumbbell Step-Up : 3 hard sets	×	×	×
Romanian Deadlift: 3 hard sets	×	×	×
Hip Thrust: 3 hard sets	×	×	×

NOTES:

WORKOUT 2: PUSH AND CORE			
EXERCISES	**SETS**		
Barbell Bench Press: Warm-up and 3 hard sets	×	×	×
Seated Dumbbell Press: 3 hard sets	×	×	×
Dumbbell Bench Press: 3 hard sets	×	×	×
Dumbbell Side Lateral Raise: 3 hard sets	×	×	×
Plank: 3 hard sets			

NOTES:

WORKOUT 3: PULL			
EXERCISES	**SETS**		
Barbell Deadlift: Warm-up and 3 hard sets	×	×	×
Chin-Up: 3 hard sets	×	×	×
Lat Pulldown (Close-Grip): 3 hard sets	×	×	×
Barbell Curl: 3 hard sets	×	×	×

NOTES:

WORKOUT 4: UPPER BODY AND CORE			
EXERCISES	SETS		
Seated Dumbbell Press: Warm-up and 3 hard sets	×	×	×
Dumbbell Bench Press: 3 hard sets	×	×	×
Dumbbell Rear Lateral Raise (Bent-Over): 3 hard sets	×	×	×
Triceps Pushdown: 3 hard sets	×	×	×
Abdominal Rollout: 3 hard sets			

NOTES:
_____
_____
_____

WORKOUT 5: LOWER BODY (LEGS AND GLUTES)			
EXERCISES	SETS		
Barbell Squat: Warm-up and 3 hard sets	×	×	×
Barbell Step-Up: 3 hard sets	×	×	×
Leg Curl (Lying or Seated)*: 3 hard sets	×	×	×
Glute Blaster: 3 hard sets	×	×	×

NOTES:
_____
_____
_____

5-DAY ROUTINE | PHASE 3 | WEEK 20

WORKOUT 1: LOWER BODY (LEGS AND GLUTES)

EXERCISES	SETS		
Barbell Squat: Warm-up and 3 hard sets	×	×	×
Dumbbell Step-Up : 3 hard sets	×	×	×
Romanian Deadlift: 3 hard sets	×	×	×
Hip Thrust: 3 hard sets	×	×	×

NOTES:

WORKOUT 2: PUSH AND CORE

EXERCISES	SETS		
Barbell Bench Press: Warm-up and 3 hard sets	×	×	×
Seated Dumbbell Press: 3 hard sets	×	×	×
Dumbbell Bench Press: 3 hard sets	×	×	×
Dumbbell Side Lateral Raise: 3 hard sets	×	×	×
Plank: 3 hard sets			

NOTES:

WORKOUT 3: PULL

EXERCISES	SETS		
Barbell Deadlift: Warm-up and 3 hard sets	×	×	×
Chin-Up: 3 hard sets	×	×	×
Lat Pulldown (Close-Grip): 3 hard sets	×	×	×
Barbell Curl: 3 hard sets	×	×	×

NOTES:

WORKOUT 4: UPPER BODY AND CORE			
EXERCISES	**SETS**		
Seated Dumbbell Press: Warm-up and 3 hard sets	×	×	×
Dumbbell Bench Press: 3 hard sets	×	×	×
Dumbbell Rear Lateral Raise (Bent-Over): 3 hard sets	×	×	×
Triceps Pushdown: 3 hard sets	×	×	×
Abdominal Rollout: 3 hard sets			

NOTES:

_____

_____

_____

WORKOUT 5: LOWER BODY (LEGS AND GLUTES)			
EXERCISES	**SETS**		
Barbell Squat: Warm-up and 3 hard sets	×	×	×
Barbell Step-Up: 3 hard sets	×	×	×
Leg Curl (Lying or Seated)*: 3 hard sets	×	×	×
Glute Blaster: 3 hard sets	×	×	×

NOTES:

_____

_____

_____

5-DAY ROUTINE	PHASE 3	WEEK 21

WORKOUT 1: LOWER BODY (LEGS AND GLUTES)

EXERCISES	SETS		
Barbell Squat: Warm-up and 3 hard sets	×	×	×
Dumbbell Step-Up : 3 hard sets	×	×	×
Romanian Deadlift: 3 hard sets	×	×	×
Hip Thrust: 3 hard sets	×	×	×

NOTES:

WORKOUT 2: PUSH AND CORE

EXERCISES	SETS		
Barbell Bench Press: Warm-up and 3 hard sets	×	×	×
Seated Dumbbell Press: 3 hard sets	×	×	×
Dumbbell Bench Press: 3 hard sets	×	×	×
Dumbbell Side Lateral Raise: 3 hard sets	×	×	×
Plank: 3 hard sets			

NOTES:

WORKOUT 3: PULL

EXERCISES	SETS		
Barbell Deadlift: Warm-up and 3 hard sets	×	×	×
Chin-Up: 3 hard sets	×	×	×
Lat Pulldown (Close-Grip): 3 hard sets	×	×	×
Barbell Curl: 3 hard sets	×	×	×

NOTES:

WORKOUT 4: UPPER BODY AND CORE			
EXERCISES	**SETS**		
Seated Dumbbell Press: Warm-up and 3 hard sets	×	×	×
Dumbbell Bench Press: 3 hard sets	×	×	×
Dumbbell Rear Lateral Raise (Bent-Over): 3 hard sets	×	×	×
Triceps Pushdown: 3 hard sets	×	×	×
Abdominal Rollout: 3 hard sets			

NOTES:

_____

_____

_____

WORKOUT 5: LOWER BODY (LEGS AND GLUTES)			
EXERCISES	**SETS**		
Barbell Squat: Warm-up and 3 hard sets	×	×	×
Barbell Step-Up: 3 hard sets	×	×	×
Leg Curl (Lying or Seated)*: 3 hard sets	×	×	×
Glute Blaster: 3 hard sets	×	×	×

NOTES:

_____

_____

_____

5-DAY ROUTINE	PHASE 3	WEEK 22

WORKOUT 1: LOWER BODY (LEGS AND GLUTES)			
EXERCISES	**SETS**		
Barbell Squat: Warm-up and 3 hard sets	×	×	×
Dumbbell Step-Up : 3 hard sets	×	×	×
Romanian Deadlift: 3 hard sets	×	×	×
Hip Thrust: 3 hard sets	×	×	×

NOTES:

WORKOUT 2: PUSH AND CORE			
EXERCISES	**SETS**		
Barbell Bench Press: Warm-up and 3 hard sets	×	×	×
Seated Dumbbell Press: 3 hard sets	×	×	×
Dumbbell Bench Press: 3 hard sets	×	×	×
Dumbbell Side Lateral Raise: 3 hard sets	×	×	×
Plank: 3 hard sets			

NOTES:

WORKOUT 3: PULL			
EXERCISES	**SETS**		
Barbell Deadlift: Warm-up and 3 hard sets	×	×	×
Chin-Up: 3 hard sets	×	×	×
Lat Pulldown (Close-Grip): 3 hard sets	×	×	×
Barbell Curl: 3 hard sets	×	×	×

NOTES:

WORKOUT 4: UPPER BODY AND CORE			
EXERCISES	SETS		
Seated Dumbbell Press: Warm-up and 3 hard sets	×	×	×
Dumbbell Bench Press: 3 hard sets	×	×	×
Dumbbell Rear Lateral Raise (Bent-Over): 3 hard sets	×	×	×
Triceps Pushdown: 3 hard sets	×	×	×
Abdominal Rollout: 3 hard sets			

NOTES:

_____

_____

_____

WORKOUT 5: LOWER BODY (LEGS AND GLUTES)			
EXERCISES	SETS		
Barbell Squat: Warm-up and 3 hard sets	×	×	×
Barbell Step-Up: 3 hard sets	×	×	×
Leg Curl (Lying or Seated)*: 3 hard sets	×	×	×
Glute Blaster: 3 hard sets	×	×	×

NOTES:

_____

_____

_____

5-DAY ROUTINE	PHASE 3	WEEK 23

WORKOUT 1: LOWER BODY (LEGS AND GLUTES)

EXERCISES	SETS		
Barbell Squat: Warm-up and 3 hard sets	×	×	×
Dumbbell Step-Up : 3 hard sets	×	×	×
Romanian Deadlift: 3 hard sets	×	×	×
Hip Thrust: 3 hard sets	×	×	×

NOTES:

WORKOUT 2: PUSH AND CORE

EXERCISES	SETS		
Barbell Bench Press: Warm-up and 3 hard sets	×	×	×
Seated Dumbbell Press: 3 hard sets	×	×	×
Dumbbell Bench Press: 3 hard sets	×	×	×
Dumbbell Side Lateral Raise: 3 hard sets	×	×	×
Plank: 3 hard sets			

NOTES:

WORKOUT 3: PULL

EXERCISES	SETS		
Barbell Deadlift: Warm-up and 3 hard sets	×	×	×
Chin-Up: 3 hard sets	×	×	×
Lat Pulldown (Close-Grip): 3 hard sets	×	×	×
Barbell Curl: 3 hard sets	×	×	×

NOTES:

WORKOUT 4: UPPER BODY AND CORE			
EXERCISES	**SETS**		
Seated Dumbbell Press: Warm-up and 3 hard sets	×	×	×
Dumbbell Bench Press: 3 hard sets	×	×	×
Dumbbell Rear Lateral Raise (Bent-Over): 3 hard sets	×	×	×
Triceps Pushdown: 3 hard sets	×	×	×
Abdominal Rollout: 3 hard sets			

NOTES:

_____

_____

_____

WORKOUT 5: LOWER BODY (LEGS AND GLUTES)			
EXERCISES	**SETS**		
Barbell Squat: Warm-up and 3 hard sets	×	×	×
Barbell Step-Up: 3 hard sets	×	×	×
Leg Curl (Lying or Seated)*: 3 hard sets	×	×	×
Glute Blaster: 3 hard sets	×	×	×

NOTES:

_____

_____

_____

5-DAY ROUTINE	PHASE 3	WEEK 24

WORKOUT 1: LOWER BODY (LEGS AND GLUTES)

EXERCISES	SETS		
Barbell Squat: Warm-up and 3 hard sets	×	×	×
Dumbbell Step-Up : 3 hard sets	×	×	×
Romanian Deadlift: 3 hard sets	×	×	×
Hip Thrust: 3 hard sets	×	×	×

NOTES:

WORKOUT 2: PUSH AND CORE

EXERCISES	SETS		
Barbell Bench Press: Warm-up and 3 hard sets	×	×	×
Seated Dumbbell Press: 3 hard sets	×	×	×
Dumbbell Bench Press: 3 hard sets	×	×	×
Dumbbell Side Lateral Raise: 3 hard sets	×	×	×
Plank: 3 hard sets			

NOTES:

WORKOUT 3: PULL

EXERCISES	SETS		
Barbell Deadlift: Warm-up and 3 hard sets	×	×	×
Chin-Up: 3 hard sets	×	×	×
Lat Pulldown (Close-Grip): 3 hard sets	×	×	×
Barbell Curl: 3 hard sets	×	×	×

NOTES:

WORKOUT 4: UPPER BODY AND CORE			
EXERCISES	**SETS**		
Seated Dumbbell Press: Warm-up and 3 hard sets	×	×	×
Dumbbell Bench Press: 3 hard sets	×	×	×
Dumbbell Rear Lateral Raise (Bent-Over): 3 hard sets	×	×	×
Triceps Pushdown: 3 hard sets	×	×	×
Abdominal Rollout: 3 hard sets			

NOTES:

_____

_____

_____

WORKOUT 5: LOWER BODY (LEGS AND GLUTES)			
EXERCISES	**SETS**		
Barbell Squat: Warm-up and 3 hard sets	×	×	×
Barbell Step-Up: 3 hard sets	×	×	×
Leg Curl (Lying or Seated)*: 3 hard sets	×	×	×
Glute Blaster: 3 hard sets	×	×	×

NOTES:

_____

_____

_____

5-DAY ROUTINE	PHASE 3	WEEK 25

WORKOUT 1: LOWER BODY (LEGS AND GLUTES)

EXERCISES	SETS		
Barbell Squat: Warm-up and 3 hard sets	×	×	×
Dumbbell Step-Up : 3 hard sets	×	×	×
Romanian Deadlift: 3 hard sets	×	×	×
Hip Thrust: 3 hard sets	×	×	×

NOTES:

WORKOUT 2: PUSH AND CORE

EXERCISES	SETS		
Barbell Bench Press: Warm-up and 3 hard sets	×	×	×
Seated Dumbbell Press: 3 hard sets	×	×	×
Dumbbell Bench Press: 3 hard sets	×	×	×
Dumbbell Side Lateral Raise: 3 hard sets	×	×	×
Plank: 3 hard sets			

NOTES:

WORKOUT 3: PULL

EXERCISES	SETS		
Barbell Deadlift: Warm-up and 3 hard sets	×	×	×
Chin-Up: 3 hard sets	×	×	×
Lat Pulldown (Close-Grip): 3 hard sets	×	×	×
Barbell Curl: 3 hard sets	×	×	×

NOTES:

WORKOUT 4: UPPER BODY AND CORE			
EXERCISES	**SETS**		
Seated Dumbbell Press: Warm-up and 3 hard sets	×	×	×
Dumbbell Bench Press: 3 hard sets	×	×	×
Dumbbell Rear Lateral Raise (Bent-Over): 3 hard sets	×	×	×
Triceps Pushdown: 3 hard sets	×	×	×
Abdominal Rollout: 3 hard sets			

NOTES:

_____

_____

_____

WORKOUT 5: LOWER BODY (LEGS AND GLUTES)			
EXERCISES	**SETS**		
Barbell Squat: Warm-up and 3 hard sets	×	×	×
Barbell Step-Up: 3 hard sets	×	×	×
Leg Curl (Lying or Seated)*: 3 hard sets	×	×	×
Glute Blaster: 3 hard sets	×	×	×

NOTES:

_____

_____

_____

5-DAY ROUTINE	PHASE 3	WEEK 26

WORKOUT 1: LOWER BODY (LEGS AND GLUTES)			
EXERCISES	**SETS**		
Barbell Squat: Warm-up and 3 hard sets	×	×	×
Dumbbell Step-Up : 3 hard sets	×	×	×
Romanian Deadlift: 3 hard sets	×	×	×
Hip Thrust: 3 hard sets	×	×	×

NOTES:

WORKOUT 2: PUSH AND CORE			
EXERCISES	**SETS**		
Barbell Bench Press: Warm-up and 3 hard sets	×	×	×
Seated Dumbbell Press: 3 hard sets	×	×	×
Dumbbell Bench Press: 3 hard sets	×	×	×
Dumbbell Side Lateral Raise: 3 hard sets	×	×	×
Plank: 3 hard sets			

NOTES:

WORKOUT 3: PULL			
EXERCISES	**SETS**		
Barbell Deadlift: Warm-up and 3 hard sets	×	×	×
Chin-Up: 3 hard sets	×	×	×
Lat Pulldown (Close-Grip): 3 hard sets	×	×	×
Barbell Curl: 3 hard sets	×	×	×

NOTES:

WORKOUT 4: UPPER BODY AND CORE			
EXERCISES	**SETS**		
Seated Dumbbell Press: Warm-up and 3 hard sets	×	×	×
Dumbbell Bench Press: 3 hard sets	×	×	×
Dumbbell Rear Lateral Raise (Bent-Over): 3 hard sets	×	×	×
Triceps Pushdown: 3 hard sets	×	×	×
Abdominal Rollout: 3 hard sets			

NOTES:

_____

_____

_____

WORKOUT 5: LOWER BODY (LEGS AND GLUTES)			
EXERCISES	**SETS**		
Barbell Squat: Warm-up and 3 hard sets	×	×	×
Barbell Step-Up: 3 hard sets	×	×	×
Leg Curl (Lying or Seated)*: 3 hard sets	×	×	×
Glute Blaster: 3 hard sets	×	×	×

NOTES:

_____

_____

_____

5-DAY ROUTINE	DELOAD	WEEK 27

WORKOUT 1: DELOAD LEGS			
EXERCISES	**SETS**		
Barbell Squat: Warm-up and 3 sets of 5 reps with last hard set weight	×	×	×
Romanian Deadlift: 3 sets of 5 reps with last hard set weight	×	×	×
Hip Thrust: 3 sets of 5 reps with last hard set weight	×	×	×

NOTES:

WORKOUT 2: DELOAD PUSH			
EXERCISES	**SETS**		
Barbell Bench Press: Warm-up and 3 sets of 5 reps with last hard set weight	×	×	×
Seated Dumbbell Press: 3 sets of 5 reps with last hard set weight	×	×	×
Dumbbell Side Lateral Raise: 3 sets of 5 reps with last hard set weight	×	×	×

NOTES:

WORKOUT 3: DELOAD PULL			
EXERCISES	**SETS**		
Barbell Deadlift: Warm-up and 3 sets of 5 reps with last hard set weight	×	×	×
Barbell Row: 3 sets of 5 reps with last hard set weight	×	×	×
Lat Pulldown (Wide-Grip): 3 sets of 5 reps with last hard set weight	×	×	×

NOTES:

4-DAY ROUTINE	PHASE 3	WEEK 19

WORKOUT 1: LOWER BODY (LEGS AND GLUTES)

EXERCISES	SETS		
Barbell Squat: Warm-up and 3 hard sets	×	×	×
Dumbbell Step-Up : 3 hard sets	×	×	×
Romanian Deadlift: 3 hard sets	×	×	×
Hip Thrust: 3 hard sets	×	×	×

NOTES:

WORKOUT 2: UPPER BODY AND CORE

EXERCISES	SETS		
Barbell Bench Press: Warm-up and 3 hard sets	×	×	×
Seated Dumbbell Press: 3 hard sets	×	×	×
Dumbbell Rear Lateral Raise (Seated): 3 hard sets	×	×	×
Triceps Pushdown: 3 hard sets	×	×	×
Abdominal Rollout: 3 hard sets			

NOTES:

WORKOUT 3: PULL			
EXERCISES	SETS		
Barbell Deadlift: Warm-up and 3 hard sets	×	×	×
Chin-Up: 3 hard sets	×	×	×
Lat Pulldown (Close-Grip): 3 hard sets	×	×	×
Barbell Curl: 3 hard sets	×	×	×

NOTES:
_____
_____
_____

WORKOUT 4: LOWER BODY (LEGS AND GLUTES)			
EXERCISES	SETS		
Barbell Squat: Warm-up and 3 hard sets	×	×	×
Barbell Step-Up: 3 hard sets	×	×	×
Leg Curl (Lying or Seated)*: 3 hard sets	×	×	×
Glute Blaster: 3 hard sets	×	×	×

NOTES:
_____
_____
_____

4-DAY ROUTINE	PHASE 3	WEEK 20

WORKOUT 1: LOWER BODY (LEGS AND GLUTES)

EXERCISES	SETS		
Barbell Squat: Warm-up and 3 hard sets	×	×	×
Dumbbell Step-Up : 3 hard sets	×	×	×
Romanian Deadlift: 3 hard sets	×	×	×
Hip Thrust: 3 hard sets	×	×	×

NOTES:

WORKOUT 2: UPPER BODY AND CORE

EXERCISES	SETS		
Barbell Bench Press: Warm-up and 3 hard sets	×	×	×
Seated Dumbbell Press: 3 hard sets	×	×	×
Dumbbell Rear Lateral Raise (Seated): 3 hard sets	×	×	×
Triceps Pushdown: 3 hard sets	×	×	×
Abdominal Rollout: 3 hard sets			

NOTES:

WORKOUT 3: PULL			
EXERCISES	**SETS**		
Barbell Deadlift: Warm-up and 3 hard sets	×	×	×
Chin-Up: 3 hard sets	×	×	×
Lat Pulldown (Close-Grip): 3 hard sets	×	×	×
Barbell Curl: 3 hard sets	×	×	×

NOTES:

_____

_____

_____

WORKOUT 4: LOWER BODY (LEGS AND GLUTES)			
EXERCISES	**SETS**		
Barbell Squat: Warm-up and 3 hard sets	×	×	×
Barbell Step-Up: 3 hard sets	×	×	×
Leg Curl (Lying or Seated)*: 3 hard sets	×	×	×
Glute Blaster: 3 hard sets	×	×	×

NOTES:

_____

_____

_____

4-DAY ROUTINE	PHASE 3	WEEK 21

WORKOUT 1: LOWER BODY (LEGS AND GLUTES)

EXERCISES	SETS		
Barbell Squat: Warm-up and 3 hard sets	×	×	×
Dumbbell Step-Up : 3 hard sets	×	×	×
Romanian Deadlift: 3 hard sets	×	×	×
Hip Thrust: 3 hard sets	×	×	×

NOTES:

WORKOUT 2: UPPER BODY AND CORE

EXERCISES	SETS		
Barbell Bench Press: Warm-up and 3 hard sets	×	×	×
Seated Dumbbell Press: 3 hard sets	×	×	×
Dumbbell Rear Lateral Raise (Seated): 3 hard sets	×	×	×
Triceps Pushdown: 3 hard sets	×	×	×
Abdominal Rollout: 3 hard sets			

NOTES:

WORKOUT 3: PULL			
EXERCISES	**SETS**		
Barbell Deadlift: Warm-up and 3 hard sets	×	×	×
Chin-Up: 3 hard sets	×	×	×
Lat Pulldown (Close-Grip): 3 hard sets	×	×	×
Barbell Curl: 3 hard sets	×	×	×

NOTES:
_____
_____
_____

WORKOUT 4: LOWER BODY (LEGS AND GLUTES)			
EXERCISES	**SETS**		
Barbell Squat: Warm-up and 3 hard sets	×	×	×
Barbell Step-Up: 3 hard sets	×	×	×
Leg Curl (Lying or Seated)*: 3 hard sets	×	×	×
Glute Blaster: 3 hard sets	×	×	×

NOTES:
_____
_____
_____

4-DAY ROUTINE	PHASE 3	WEEK 22

WORKOUT 1: LOWER BODY (LEGS AND GLUTES)			
EXERCISES	SETS		
Barbell Squat: Warm-up and 3 hard sets	×	×	×
Dumbbell Step-Up : 3 hard sets	×	×	×
Romanian Deadlift: 3 hard sets	×	×	×
Hip Thrust: 3 hard sets	×	×	×

NOTES:

WORKOUT 2: UPPER BODY AND CORE			
EXERCISES	SETS		
Barbell Bench Press: Warm-up and 3 hard sets	×	×	×
Seated Dumbbell Press: 3 hard sets	×	×	×
Dumbbell Rear Lateral Raise (Seated): 3 hard sets	×	×	×
Triceps Pushdown: 3 hard sets	×	×	×
Abdominal Rollout: 3 hard sets			

NOTES:

WORKOUT 3: PULL			
EXERCISES	**SETS**		
Barbell Deadlift: Warm-up and 3 hard sets	×	×	×
Chin-Up: 3 hard sets	×	×	×
Lat Pulldown (Close-Grip): 3 hard sets	×	×	×
Barbell Curl: 3 hard sets	×	×	×

NOTES:

WORKOUT 4: LOWER BODY (LEGS AND GLUTES)			
EXERCISES	**SETS**		
Barbell Squat: Warm-up and 3 hard sets	×	×	×
Barbell Step-Up: 3 hard sets	×	×	×
Leg Curl (Lying or Seated)*: 3 hard sets	×	×	×
Glute Blaster: 3 hard sets	×	×	×

NOTES:

4-DAY ROUTINE	PHASE 3	WEEK 23

WORKOUT 1: LOWER BODY (LEGS AND GLUTES)

EXERCISES	SETS		
Barbell Squat: Warm-up and 3 hard sets	×	×	×
Dumbbell Step-Up : 3 hard sets	×	×	×
Romanian Deadlift: 3 hard sets	×	×	×
Hip Thrust: 3 hard sets	×	×	×

NOTES:

_____

_____

WORKOUT 2: UPPER BODY AND CORE

EXERCISES	SETS		
Barbell Bench Press: Warm-up and 3 hard sets	×	×	×
Seated Dumbbell Press: 3 hard sets	×	×	×
Dumbbell Rear Lateral Raise (Seated): 3 hard sets	×	×	×
Triceps Pushdown: 3 hard sets	×	×	×
Abdominal Rollout: 3 hard sets			

NOTES:

_____

_____

WORKOUT 3: PULL			
EXERCISES	**SETS**		
Barbell Deadlift: Warm-up and 3 hard sets	×	×	×
Chin-Up: 3 hard sets	×	×	×
Lat Pulldown (Close-Grip): 3 hard sets	×	×	×
Barbell Curl: 3 hard sets	×	×	×

NOTES:

_____

_____

_____

WORKOUT 4: LOWER BODY (LEGS AND GLUTES)			
EXERCISES	**SETS**		
Barbell Squat: Warm-up and 3 hard sets	×	×	×
Barbell Step-Up: 3 hard sets	×	×	×
Leg Curl (Lying or Seated)*: 3 hard sets	×	×	×
Glute Blaster: 3 hard sets	×	×	×

NOTES:

_____

_____

_____

| 4-DAY ROUTINE | PHASE 3 | WEEK 24 |

WORKOUT 1: LOWER BODY (LEGS AND GLUTES)

EXERCISES	SETS		
Barbell Squat: Warm-up and 3 hard sets	×	×	×
Dumbbell Step-Up : 3 hard sets	×	×	×
Romanian Deadlift: 3 hard sets	×	×	×
Hip Thrust: 3 hard sets	×	×	×

NOTES:

_____

_____

WORKOUT 2: UPPER BODY AND CORE

EXERCISES	SETS		
Barbell Bench Press: Warm-up and 3 hard sets	×	×	×
Seated Dumbbell Press: 3 hard sets	×	×	×
Dumbbell Rear Lateral Raise (Seated): 3 hard sets	×	×	×
Triceps Pushdown: 3 hard sets	×	×	×
Abdominal Rollout: 3 hard sets			

NOTES:

_____

_____

WORKOUT 3: PULL			
EXERCISES	**SETS**		
Barbell Deadlift: Warm-up and 3 hard sets	×	×	×
Chin-Up: 3 hard sets	×	×	×
Lat Pulldown (Close-Grip): 3 hard sets	×	×	×
Barbell Curl: 3 hard sets	×	×	×

NOTES:

WORKOUT 4: LOWER BODY (LEGS AND GLUTES)			
EXERCISES	**SETS**		
Barbell Squat: Warm-up and 3 hard sets	×	×	×
Barbell Step-Up: 3 hard sets	×	×	×
Leg Curl (Lying or Seated)*: 3 hard sets	×	×	×
Glute Blaster: 3 hard sets	×	×	×

NOTES:

| 4-DAY ROUTINE | PHASE 3 | WEEK 25 |

WORKOUT 1: LOWER BODY (LEGS AND GLUTES)

EXERCISES	SETS		
Barbell Squat: Warm-up and 3 hard sets	×	×	×
Dumbbell Step-Up : 3 hard sets	×	×	×
Romanian Deadlift: 3 hard sets	×	×	×
Hip Thrust: 3 hard sets	×	×	×

NOTES:

WORKOUT 2: UPPER BODY AND CORE

EXERCISES	SETS		
Barbell Bench Press: Warm-up and 3 hard sets	×	×	×
Seated Dumbbell Press: 3 hard sets	×	×	×
Dumbbell Rear Lateral Raise (Seated): 3 hard sets	×	×	×
Triceps Pushdown: 3 hard sets	×	×	×
Abdominal Rollout: 3 hard sets			

NOTES:

WORKOUT 3: PULL			
EXERCISES	**SETS**		
Barbell Deadlift: Warm-up and 3 hard sets	×	×	×
Chin-Up: 3 hard sets	×	×	×
Lat Pulldown (Close-Grip): 3 hard sets	×	×	×
Barbell Curl: 3 hard sets	×	×	×

NOTES:
_____
_____
_____

WORKOUT 4: LOWER BODY (LEGS AND GLUTES)			
EXERCISES	**SETS**		
Barbell Squat: Warm-up and 3 hard sets	×	×	×
Barbell Step-Up: 3 hard sets	×	×	×
Leg Curl (Lying or Seated)*: 3 hard sets	×	×	×
Glute Blaster: 3 hard sets	×	×	×

NOTES:
_____
_____
_____

4-DAY ROUTINE	PHASE 3	WEEK 26

WORKOUT 1: LOWER BODY (LEGS AND GLUTES)

EXERCISES	SETS		
Barbell Squat: Warm-up and 3 hard sets	×	×	×
Dumbbell Step-Up : 3 hard sets	×	×	×
Romanian Deadlift: 3 hard sets	×	×	×
Hip Thrust: 3 hard sets	×	×	×

NOTES:

WORKOUT 2: UPPER BODY AND CORE

EXERCISES	SETS		
Barbell Bench Press: Warm-up and 3 hard sets	×	×	×
Seated Dumbbell Press: 3 hard sets	×	×	×
Dumbbell Rear Lateral Raise (Seated): 3 hard sets	×	×	×
Triceps Pushdown: 3 hard sets	×	×	×
Abdominal Rollout: 3 hard sets			

NOTES:

WORKOUT 3: PULL			
EXERCISES	**SETS**		
Barbell Deadlift: Warm-up and 3 hard sets	×	×	×
Chin-Up: 3 hard sets	×	×	×
Lat Pulldown (Close-Grip): 3 hard sets	×	×	×
Barbell Curl: 3 hard sets	×	×	×

NOTES:

_____

_____

_____

WORKOUT 4: LOWER BODY (LEGS AND GLUTES)			
EXERCISES	**SETS**		
Barbell Squat: Warm-up and 3 hard sets	×	×	×
Barbell Step-Up: 3 hard sets	×	×	×
Leg Curl (Lying or Seated)*: 3 hard sets	×	×	×
Glute Blaster: 3 hard sets	×	×	×

NOTES:

_____

_____

_____

4-DAY ROUTINE	DELOAD	WEEK 27

WORKOUT 1: DELOAD LEGS

EXERCISES	SETS		
Barbell Squat: Warm-up and 3 sets of 5 reps with last hard set weight	×	×	×
Romanian Deadlift: 3 sets of 5 reps with last hard set weight	×	×	×
Hip Thrust: 3 sets of 5 reps with last hard set weight	×	×	×

NOTES:

WORKOUT 2: DELOAD PUSH

EXERCISES	SETS		
Barbell Bench Press: Warm-up and 3 sets of 5 reps with last hard set weight	×	×	×
Seated Dumbbell Press: 3 sets of 5 reps with last hard set weight	×	×	×
Dumbbell Bench Press: 3 sets of 5 reps with last hard set weight	×	×	×

NOTES:

WORKOUT 3: DELOAD PULL

EXERCISES	SETS		
Barbell Deadlift: Warm-up and 3 sets of 5 reps with last hard set weight	×	×	×
Barbell Row: 3 sets of 5 reps with last hard set weight	×	×	×
Lat Pulldown (Wide-Grip): 3 sets of 5 reps with last hard set weight	×	×	×

NOTES:

3-DAY ROUTINE	PHASE 3	WEEK 19

WORKOUT 1: LOWER BODY (LEGS AND GLUTES)

EXERCISES	SETS		
Barbell Squat: Warm-up and 3 hard sets	×	×	×
Dumbbell Step-Up : 3 hard sets	×	×	×
Romanian Deadlift: 3 hard sets	×	×	×
Hip Thrust: 3 hard sets	×	×	×

NOTES:

WORKOUT 2: UPPER BODY AND CORE

EXERCISES	SETS		
Barbell Bench Press: Warm-up and 3 hard sets	×	×	×
Seated Dumbbell Press: 3 hard sets	×	×	×
Dumbbell Side Lateral Raise: 3 hard sets	×	×	×
Triceps Pushdown: 3 hard sets	×	×	×
Plank: 3 hard sets			

NOTES:

WORKOUT 3: LOWER BODY AND PULL (LEGS AND BACK)

EXERCISES	SETS		
Barbell Squat: Warm-up and 3 hard sets	×	×	×
Barbell Deadlift: Warm-up and 3 hard sets	×	×	×
Barbell Row: 3 hard sets	×	×	×
Lat Pulldown (Wide-Grip): 3 hard sets	×	×	×
E-Z Bar Curl: 3 hard sets	×	×	×

NOTES:

3-DAY ROUTINE	PHASE 3	WEEK 20

WORKOUT 1: LOWER BODY (LEGS AND GLUTES)

EXERCISES	SETS		
Barbell Squat: Warm-up and 3 hard sets	×	×	×
Dumbbell Step-Up : 3 hard sets	×	×	×
Romanian Deadlift: 3 hard sets	×	×	×
Hip Thrust: 3 hard sets	×	×	×

NOTES:

EXERCISES

EXERCISES	SETS		
Barbell Bench Press: Warm-up and 3 hard sets	×	×	×
Seated Dumbbell Press: 3 hard sets	×	×	×
Dumbbell Side Lateral Raise: 3 hard sets	×	×	×
Triceps Pushdown: 3 hard sets	×	×	×
Plank: 3 hard sets			

NOTES:

WORKOUT 3: LOWER BODY AND PULL (LEGS AND BACK)

EXERCISES	SETS		
Barbell Squat: Warm-up and 3 hard sets	×	×	×
Barbell Deadlift: Warm-up and 3 hard sets	×	×	×
Barbell Row: 3 hard sets	×	×	×
Lat Pulldown (Wide-Grip): 3 hard sets	×	×	×
E-Z Bar Curl: 3 hard sets	×	×	×

NOTES:

3-DAY ROUTINE	PHASE 3	WEEK 21

WORKOUT 1: LOWER BODY (LEGS AND GLUTES)

EXERCISES	SETS		
Barbell Squat: Warm-up and 3 hard sets	×	×	×
Dumbbell Step-Up : 3 hard sets	×	×	×
Romanian Deadlift: 3 hard sets	×	×	×
Hip Thrust: 3 hard sets	×	×	×

NOTES:

WORKOUT 2: UPPER BODY AND CORE

EXERCISES	SETS		
Barbell Bench Press: Warm-up and 3 hard sets	×	×	×
Seated Dumbbell Press: 3 hard sets	×	×	×
Dumbbell Side Lateral Raise: 3 hard sets	×	×	×
Triceps Pushdown: 3 hard sets	×	×	×
Plank: 3 hard sets			

NOTES:

WORKOUT 3: LOWER BODY AND PULL (LEGS AND BACK)

EXERCISES	SETS		
Barbell Squat: Warm-up and 3 hard sets	×	×	×
Barbell Deadlift: Warm-up and 3 hard sets	×	×	×
Barbell Row: 3 hard sets	×	×	×
Lat Pulldown (Wide-Grip): 3 hard sets	×	×	×
E-Z Bar Curl: 3 hard sets	×	×	×

NOTES:

3-DAY ROUTINE	PHASE 3	WEEK 22

WORKOUT 1: LOWER BODY (LEGS AND GLUTES)

EXERCISES	SETS		
Barbell Squat: Warm-up and 3 hard sets	×	×	×
Dumbbell Step-Up : 3 hard sets	×	×	×
Romanian Deadlift: 3 hard sets	×	×	×
Hip Thrust: 3 hard sets	×	×	×

NOTES:

EXERCISES

EXERCISES	SETS		
Barbell Bench Press: Warm-up and 3 hard sets	×	×	×
Seated Dumbbell Press: 3 hard sets	×	×	×
Dumbbell Side Lateral Raise: 3 hard sets	×	×	×
Triceps Pushdown: 3 hard sets	×	×	×
Plank: 3 hard sets			

NOTES:

WORKOUT 3: LOWER BODY AND PULL (LEGS AND BACK)

EXERCISES	SETS		
Barbell Squat: Warm-up and 3 hard sets	×	×	×
Barbell Deadlift: Warm-up and 3 hard sets	×	×	×
Barbell Row: 3 hard sets	×	×	×
Lat Pulldown (Wide-Grip): 3 hard sets	×	×	×
E-Z Bar Curl: 3 hard sets	×	×	×

NOTES:

3-DAY ROUTINE	PHASE 3	WEEK 23

WORKOUT 1: LOWER BODY (LEGS AND GLUTES)

EXERCISES	SETS		
Barbell Squat: Warm-up and 3 hard sets	×	×	×
Dumbbell Step-Up : 3 hard sets	×	×	×
Romanian Deadlift: 3 hard sets	×	×	×
Hip Thrust: 3 hard sets	×	×	×

NOTES:

WORKOUT 2: UPPER BODY AND CORE

EXERCISES	SETS		
Barbell Bench Press: Warm-up and 3 hard sets	×	×	×
Seated Dumbbell Press: 3 hard sets	×	×	×
Dumbbell Side Lateral Raise: 3 hard sets	×	×	×
Triceps Pushdown: 3 hard sets	×	×	×
Plank: 3 hard sets			

NOTES:

WORKOUT 3: LOWER BODY AND PULL (LEGS AND BACK)

EXERCISES	SETS		
Barbell Squat: Warm-up and 3 hard sets	×	×	×
Barbell Deadlift: Warm-up and 3 hard sets	×	×	×
Barbell Row: 3 hard sets	×	×	×
Lat Pulldown (Wide-Grip): 3 hard sets	×	×	×
E-Z Bar Curl: 3 hard sets	×	×	×

NOTES:

| 3-DAY ROUTINE | PHASE 3 | WEEK 24 |

WORKOUT 1: LOWER BODY (LEGS AND GLUTES)

EXERCISES	SETS		
Barbell Squat: Warm-up and 3 hard sets	×	×	×
Dumbbell Step-Up : 3 hard sets	×	×	×
Romanian Deadlift: 3 hard sets	×	×	×
Hip Thrust: 3 hard sets	×	×	×

NOTES:

EXERCISES

EXERCISES	SETS		
Barbell Bench Press: Warm-up and 3 hard sets	×	×	×
Seated Dumbbell Press: 3 hard sets	×	×	×
Dumbbell Side Lateral Raise: 3 hard sets	×	×	×
Triceps Pushdown: 3 hard sets	×	×	×
Plank: 3 hard sets			

NOTES:

WORKOUT 3: LOWER BODY AND PULL (LEGS AND BACK)

EXERCISES	SETS		
Barbell Squat: Warm-up and 3 hard sets	×	×	×
Barbell Deadlift: Warm-up and 3 hard sets	×	×	×
Barbell Row: 3 hard sets	×	×	×
Lat Pulldown (Wide-Grip): 3 hard sets	×	×	×
E-Z Bar Curl: 3 hard sets	×	×	×

NOTES:

3-DAY ROUTINE	PHASE 3	WEEK 25

WORKOUT 1: LOWER BODY (LEGS AND GLUTES)

EXERCISES	SETS		
Barbell Squat: Warm-up and 3 hard sets	×	×	×
Dumbbell Step-Up : 3 hard sets	×	×	×
Romanian Deadlift: 3 hard sets	×	×	×
Hip Thrust: 3 hard sets	×	×	×

NOTES:

WORKOUT 2: UPPER BODY AND CORE

EXERCISES	SETS		
Barbell Bench Press: Warm-up and 3 hard sets	×	×	×
Seated Dumbbell Press: 3 hard sets	×	×	×
Dumbbell Side Lateral Raise: 3 hard sets	×	×	×
Triceps Pushdown: 3 hard sets	×	×	×
Plank: 3 hard sets			

NOTES:

WORKOUT 3: LOWER BODY AND PULL (LEGS AND BACK)

EXERCISES	SETS		
Barbell Squat: Warm-up and 3 hard sets	×	×	×
Barbell Deadlift: Warm-up and 3 hard sets	×	×	×
Barbell Row: 3 hard sets	×	×	×
Lat Pulldown (Wide-Grip): 3 hard sets	×	×	×
E-Z Bar Curl: 3 hard sets	×	×	×

NOTES:

3-DAY ROUTINE	PHASE 3	WEEK 26

WORKOUT 1: LOWER BODY (LEGS AND GLUTES)

EXERCISES	SETS		
Barbell Squat: Warm-up and 3 hard sets	×	×	×
Dumbbell Step-Up : 3 hard sets	×	×	×
Romanian Deadlift: 3 hard sets	×	×	×
Hip Thrust: 3 hard sets	×	×	×

NOTES:

_____

_____

_____

EXERCISES

EXERCISES	SETS		
Barbell Bench Press: Warm-up and 3 hard sets	×	×	×
Seated Dumbbell Press: 3 hard sets	×	×	×
Dumbbell Side Lateral Raise: 3 hard sets	×	×	×
Triceps Pushdown: 3 hard sets	×	×	×
Plank: 3 hard sets			

NOTES:

_____

_____

_____

WORKOUT 3: LOWER BODY AND PULL (LEGS AND BACK)

EXERCISES	SETS		
Barbell Squat: Warm-up and 3 hard sets	×	×	×
Barbell Deadlift: Warm-up and 3 hard sets	×	×	×
Barbell Row: 3 hard sets	×	×	×
Lat Pulldown (Wide-Grip): 3 hard sets	×	×	×
E-Z Bar Curl: 3 hard sets	×	×	×

NOTES:

_____

_____

_____

3-DAY ROUTINE	DELOAD	WEEK 27

WORKOUT 1: DELOAD LEGS

EXERCISES	SETS		
Barbell Squat: Warm-up and 3 sets of 5 reps with last hard set weight	×	×	×
Romanian Deadlift: 3 sets of 5 reps with last hard set weight	×	×	×
Hip Thrust: 3 sets of 5 reps with last hard set weight	×	×	×

NOTES:

_____

_____

_____

WORKOUT 2: DELOAD PUSH

EXERCISES	SETS		
Barbell Bench Press: Warm-up and 3 sets of 5 reps with last hard set weight	×	×	×
Seated Dumbbell Press: 3 sets of 5 reps with last hard set weight	×	×	×
Dumbbell Bench Press: 3 sets of 5 reps with last hard set weight	×	×	×

NOTES:

_____

_____

_____

WORKOUT 3: DELOAD PULL

EXERCISES	SETS		
Barbell Deadlift: Warm-up and 3 sets of 5 reps with last hard set weight	×	×	×
Barbell Row: 3 sets of 5 reps with last hard set weight	×	×	×
Lat Pulldown (Wide-Grip): 3 sets of 5 reps with last hard set weight	×	×	×

NOTES:

_____

_____

_____

Put a fork in it. Phase 3 is done!

You're that much closer to the body you really want, and by now, your hard work is paying some serious dividends. Just look at your pictures and measurements!
(You ARE taking them, right? If not, get started now! It's not too late.)

The next phase is going to be a bit tougher than the last, but you're up to it. As you'll see, I'm changing the order of the exercises a bit so you can experience all the major compound exercises at the beginning of your workouts, when you're freshest. (This is a great way to speed up progress on any given exercise, by the way.)

As usual, before you march off to set new PRs in Phase 4, let's take new measurements and pictures!

First, take the following body measurements first thing in the morning, nude, after using the bathroom and before eating or drinking anything:

1. Weight

2. Waist circumference

3. OPTIONAL: Hip circumference

4. OPTIONAL: Upper-leg circumference

5. OPTIONAL: Flexed arms

Then, take flexed and unflexed pictures from the front, back, and sides, and store them in an album or folder that you can easily locate later.

Remember to show as much skin as you feel comfortable with. The more the better because it will give you the best idea of how your body is responding to the program.

Also, if you haven't shared your results on social media yet, now's the perfect time to post about them and inspire your friends and family! And be sure to include the #thinnerleanerstronger hashtag so that other people looking for encouragement will be able to find you and follow along.

──────────

Here's how we can connect:
Facebook: www.facebook.com/muscleforlifefitness
Instagram: www.instagram.com/muscleforlifefitness
YouTube: www.youtube.com/muscleforlifefitness
Twitter: www.twitter.com/muscleforlife

Tally-ho!

WHEN A GREAT SHIP IS IN HARBOR AND MOORED, IT IS SAFE. BUT THAT IS NOT WHAT GREAT SHIPS ARE BUILT FOR.

—DR. CLARISSA PINKOLA ESTÉS

THINNER LEANER STRONGER PHASE 4

Congratulations on completing Phase 3, and welcome to Phase 4!

Can you believe that you've reached the halfway point in the challenge? That you can now say that you've been on point with your diet and exercise for six straight months?

Pretty cool, right? Cheers—here's to six more!

I have some more good news, too:

You've now introduced your body to and performed all of the program's major exercises, which is the hardest part to learn. From here on out, there will be some new movements, but getting comfortable with the big, compound lifts is a major milestone, so great job!

All you have to do now is continue showing up to put in the work, and keep following your meal plan, and your body composition will continue to get better and better. It's not going to respond as well as it did when you first started, mind you ("newbie gains" are real!), but you will enjoy slow and steady increases in your whole-body strength and muscle definition, which is the name of the game.

You may have also noticed by now that you progress more quickly on some exercises than others. This is completely normal and nothing to worry about. We all have genetic strengths and weaknesses, and as long as you push yourself to get stronger on every exercise that you do, your body will develop just fine. (And if you're worried about potentially developing muscle imbalances go to www.muscleforlife.com/muscle-imbalances to read an article I wrote on this.)

So, on the following pages, you'll find your next nine weeks of the challenge. As before, choose the split that best suits your goals and circumstances, and stick with it until you've completed this second phase.

Before you get started, though, let's reflect on the last phase.

Answer the following questions, and if you have a lot to say, jot it down so you can easily refer back to it.

→ What are three things in your diet and/or training that went particularly well in the last phase? Why?

→ What's one thing you could have done better? Why?

→ What's one thing you can do to make your next phase even better than the last?

That's it for now. Onward and upward!

| 5-DAY ROUTINE | PHASE 4 | WEEK 28 |

WORKOUT 1: LOWER BODY (LEGS AND GLUTES)

EXERCISES	SETS		
Barbell Squat: Warm-up and 3 hard sets	×	×	×
Dumbbell Lunge (Reverse): 3 hard sets	×	×	×
Leg Curl (Lying or Seated)*: 3 hard sets	×	×	×
Dumbbell Step-Up: 3 hard sets	×	×	×

NOTES:

WORKOUT 2: PUSH AND CORE

EXERCISES	SETS		
Barbell Bench Press: Warm-up and 3 hard sets	×	×	×
Arnold Dumbbell Press: 3 hard sets	×	×	×
Dumbbell Bench Press: 3 hard sets	×	×	×
Dumbbell Rear Lateral Raise (Seated): 3 hard sets	×	×	×
Abdominal Rollout: 3 hard sets			

NOTES:

WORKOUT 3: PULL

EXERCISES	SETS		
Barbell Deadlift: Warm-up and 3 hard sets	×	×	×
One-Arm Dumbbell Row: 3 hard sets	×	×	×
T-Bar Row: 3 hard sets	×	×	×
Dumbbell Hammer Curl: 3 hard sets	×	×	×

NOTES:

WORKOUT 4: UPPER BODY AND CORE			
EXERCISES	SETS		
Arnold Dumbbell Press: Warm-up and 3 hard sets	×	×	×
Close-Grip Bench Press: 3 hard sets	×	×	×
Dumbbell Side Lateral Raise: 3 hard sets	×	×	×
Seated Triceps Press: 3 hard sets	×	×	×
Crunch: 3 hard sets			

NOTES:

_____

_____

_____

WORKOUT 5: LOWER BODY (LEGS AND GLUTES)			
EXERCISES	SETS		
Barbell Front Squat: Warm-up and 3 hard sets	×	×	×
Leg Press: 3 hard sets	×	×	×
Romanian Deadlift: 3 hard sets	×	×	×
Hip Thrust: 3 hard sets	×	×	×

NOTES:

_____

_____

_____

5-DAY ROUTINE	PHASE 4	WEEK 29

WORKOUT 1: LOWER BODY (LEGS AND GLUTES)			
EXERCISES	**SETS**		
Barbell Squat: Warm-up and 3 hard sets	×	×	×
Dumbbell Lunge (Reverse): 3 hard sets	×	×	×
Leg Curl (Lying or Seated)*: 3 hard sets	×	×	×
Dumbbell Step-Up: 3 hard sets	×	×	×

NOTES:

WORKOUT 2: PUSH AND CORE			
EXERCISES	**SETS**		
Barbell Bench Press: Warm-up and 3 hard sets	×	×	×
Arnold Dumbbell Press: 3 hard sets	×	×	×
Dumbbell Bench Press: 3 hard sets	×	×	×
Dumbbell Rear Lateral Raise (Seated): 3 hard sets	×	×	×
Abdominal Rollout: 3 hard sets			

NOTES:

WORKOUT 3: PULL			
EXERCISES	**SETS**		
Barbell Deadlift: Warm-up and 3 hard sets	×	×	×
One-Arm Dumbbell Row: 3 hard sets	×	×	×
T-Bar Row: 3 hard sets	×	×	×
Dumbbell Hammer Curl: 3 hard sets	×	×	×

NOTES:

WORKOUT 4: UPPER BODY AND CORE			
EXERCISES	**SETS**		
Arnold Dumbbell Press: Warm-up and 3 hard sets	×	×	×
Close-Grip Bench Press: 3 hard sets	×	×	×
Dumbbell Side Lateral Raise: 3 hard sets	×	×	×
Seated Triceps Press: 3 hard sets	×	×	×
Crunch: 3 hard sets			

NOTES:
_____
_____
_____

WORKOUT 5: LOWER BODY (LEGS AND GLUTES)			
EXERCISES	**SETS**		
Barbell Front Squat: Warm-up and 3 hard sets	×	×	×
Leg Press: 3 hard sets	×	×	×
Romanian Deadlift: 3 hard sets	×	×	×
Hip Thrust: 3 hard sets	×	×	×

NOTES:
_____
_____
_____

| 5-DAY ROUTINE | PHASE 4 | WEEK 30 |

WORKOUT 1: LOWER BODY (LEGS AND GLUTES)			
EXERCISES	SETS		
Barbell Squat: Warm-up and 3 hard sets	×	×	×
Dumbbell Lunge (Reverse): 3 hard sets	×	×	×
Leg Curl (Lying or Seated)*: 3 hard sets	×	×	×
Dumbbell Step-Up: 3 hard sets	×	×	×

NOTES:

WORKOUT 2: PUSH AND CORE			
EXERCISES	SETS		
Barbell Bench Press: Warm-up and 3 hard sets	×	×	×
Arnold Dumbbell Press: 3 hard sets	×	×	×
Dumbbell Bench Press: 3 hard sets	×	×	×
Dumbbell Rear Lateral Raise (Seated): 3 hard sets	×	×	×
Abdominal Rollout: 3 hard sets			

NOTES:

WORKOUT 3: PULL			
EXERCISES	SETS		
Barbell Deadlift: Warm-up and 3 hard sets	×	×	×
One-Arm Dumbbell Row: 3 hard sets	×	×	×
T-Bar Row: 3 hard sets	×	×	×
Dumbbell Hammer Curl: 3 hard sets	×	×	×

NOTES:

WORKOUT 4: UPPER BODY AND CORE			
EXERCISES	**SETS**		
Arnold Dumbbell Press: Warm-up and 3 hard sets	×	×	×
Close-Grip Bench Press: 3 hard sets	×	×	×
Dumbbell Side Lateral Raise: 3 hard sets	×	×	×
Seated Triceps Press: 3 hard sets	×	×	×
Crunch: 3 hard sets			

NOTES:

_____

_____

_____

WORKOUT 5: LOWER BODY (LEGS AND GLUTES)			
EXERCISES	**SETS**		
Barbell Front Squat: Warm-up and 3 hard sets	×	×	×
Leg Press: 3 hard sets	×	×	×
Romanian Deadlift: 3 hard sets	×	×	×
Hip Thrust: 3 hard sets	×	×	×

NOTES:

_____

_____

_____

5-DAY ROUTINE	PHASE 4	WEEK 31

WORKOUT 1: LOWER BODY (LEGS AND GLUTES)			
EXERCISES	SETS		
Barbell Squat: Warm-up and 3 hard sets	×	×	×
Dumbbell Lunge (Reverse): 3 hard sets	×	×	×
Leg Curl (Lying or Seated)*: 3 hard sets	×	×	×
Dumbbell Step-Up: 3 hard sets	×	×	×

NOTES:

WORKOUT 2: PUSH AND CORE			
EXERCISES	SETS		
Barbell Bench Press: Warm-up and 3 hard sets	×	×	×
Arnold Dumbbell Press: 3 hard sets	×	×	×
Dumbbell Bench Press: 3 hard sets	×	×	×
Dumbbell Rear Lateral Raise (Seated): 3 hard sets	×	×	×
Abdominal Rollout: 3 hard sets			

NOTES:

WORKOUT 3: PULL			
EXERCISES	SETS		
Barbell Deadlift: Warm-up and 3 hard sets	×	×	×
One-Arm Dumbbell Row: 3 hard sets	×	×	×
T-Bar Row: 3 hard sets	×	×	×
Dumbbell Hammer Curl: 3 hard sets	×	×	×

NOTES:

WORKOUT 4: UPPER BODY AND CORE			
EXERCISES	**SETS**		
Arnold Dumbbell Press: Warm-up and 3 hard sets	×	×	×
Close-Grip Bench Press: 3 hard sets	×	×	×
Dumbbell Side Lateral Raise: 3 hard sets	×	×	×
Seated Triceps Press: 3 hard sets	×	×	×
Crunch: 3 hard sets			

NOTES:

WORKOUT 5: LOWER BODY (LEGS AND GLUTES)			
EXERCISES	**SETS**		
Barbell Front Squat: Warm-up and 3 hard sets	×	×	×
Leg Press: 3 hard sets	×	×	×
Romanian Deadlift: 3 hard sets	×	×	×
Hip Thrust: 3 hard sets	×	×	×

NOTES:

5-DAY ROUTINE	PHASE 4	WEEK 32

WORKOUT 1: LOWER BODY (LEGS AND GLUTES)			
EXERCISES	**SETS**		
Barbell Squat: Warm-up and 3 hard sets	×	×	×
Dumbbell Lunge (Reverse): 3 hard sets	×	×	×
Leg Curl (Lying or Seated)*: 3 hard sets	×	×	×
Dumbbell Step-Up: 3 hard sets	×	×	×

NOTES:

WORKOUT 2: PUSH AND CORE			
EXERCISES	**SETS**		
Barbell Bench Press: Warm-up and 3 hard sets	×	×	×
Arnold Dumbbell Press: 3 hard sets	×	×	×
Dumbbell Bench Press: 3 hard sets	×	×	×
Dumbbell Rear Lateral Raise (Seated): 3 hard sets	×	×	×
Abdominal Rollout: 3 hard sets			

NOTES:

WORKOUT 3: PULL			
EXERCISES	**SETS**		
Barbell Deadlift: Warm-up and 3 hard sets	×	×	×
One-Arm Dumbbell Row: 3 hard sets	×	×	×
T-Bar Row: 3 hard sets	×	×	×
Dumbbell Hammer Curl: 3 hard sets	×	×	×

NOTES:

WORKOUT 4: UPPER BODY AND CORE			
EXERCISES	**SETS**		
Arnold Dumbbell Press: Warm-up and 3 hard sets	×	×	×
Close-Grip Bench Press: 3 hard sets	×	×	×
Dumbbell Side Lateral Raise: 3 hard sets	×	×	×
Seated Triceps Press: 3 hard sets	×	×	×
Crunch: 3 hard sets			

NOTES:

WORKOUT 5: LOWER BODY (LEGS AND GLUTES)			
EXERCISES	**SETS**		
Barbell Front Squat: Warm-up and 3 hard sets	×	×	×
Leg Press: 3 hard sets	×	×	×
Romanian Deadlift: 3 hard sets	×	×	×
Hip Thrust: 3 hard sets	×	×	×

NOTES:

5-DAY ROUTINE	PHASE 4	WEEK 33

WORKOUT 1: LOWER BODY (LEGS AND GLUTES)			
EXERCISES	**SETS**		
Barbell Squat: Warm-up and 3 hard sets	×	×	×
Dumbbell Lunge (Reverse): 3 hard sets	×	×	×
Leg Curl (Lying or Seated)*: 3 hard sets	×	×	×
Dumbbell Step-Up: 3 hard sets	×	×	×

NOTES:

WORKOUT 2: PUSH AND CORE			
EXERCISES	**SETS**		
Barbell Bench Press: Warm-up and 3 hard sets	×	×	×
Arnold Dumbbell Press: 3 hard sets	×	×	×
Dumbbell Bench Press: 3 hard sets	×	×	×
Dumbbell Rear Lateral Raise (Seated): 3 hard sets	×	×	×
Abdominal Rollout: 3 hard sets			

NOTES:

WORKOUT 3: PULL			
EXERCISES	**SETS**		
Barbell Deadlift: Warm-up and 3 hard sets	×	×	×
One-Arm Dumbbell Row: 3 hard sets	×	×	×
T-Bar Row: 3 hard sets	×	×	×
Dumbbell Hammer Curl: 3 hard sets	×	×	×

NOTES:

WORKOUT 4: UPPER BODY AND CORE			
EXERCISES	SETS		
Arnold Dumbbell Press: Warm-up and 3 hard sets	×	×	×
Close-Grip Bench Press: 3 hard sets	×	×	×
Dumbbell Side Lateral Raise: 3 hard sets	×	×	×
Seated Triceps Press: 3 hard sets	×	×	×
Crunch: 3 hard sets			

NOTES:
_____
_____
_____

WORKOUT 5: LOWER BODY (LEGS AND GLUTES)			
EXERCISES	SETS		
Barbell Front Squat: Warm-up and 3 hard sets	×	×	×
Leg Press: 3 hard sets	×	×	×
Romanian Deadlift: 3 hard sets	×	×	×
Hip Thrust: 3 hard sets	×	×	×

NOTES:
_____
_____
_____

| 5-DAY ROUTINE | PHASE 4 | WEEK 34 |

WORKOUT 1: LOWER BODY (LEGS AND GLUTES)

EXERCISES	SETS		
Barbell Squat: Warm-up and 3 hard sets	×	×	×
Dumbbell Lunge (Reverse): 3 hard sets	×	×	×
Leg Curl (Lying or Seated)*: 3 hard sets	×	×	×
Dumbbell Step-Up: 3 hard sets	×	×	×

NOTES:

WORKOUT 2: PUSH AND CORE

EXERCISES	SETS		
Barbell Bench Press: Warm-up and 3 hard sets	×	×	×
Arnold Dumbbell Press: 3 hard sets	×	×	×
Dumbbell Bench Press: 3 hard sets	×	×	×
Dumbbell Rear Lateral Raise (Seated): 3 hard sets	×	×	×
Abdominal Rollout: 3 hard sets			

NOTES:

WORKOUT 3: PULL

EXERCISES	SETS		
Barbell Deadlift: Warm-up and 3 hard sets	×	×	×
One-Arm Dumbbell Row: 3 hard sets	×	×	×
T-Bar Row: 3 hard sets	×	×	×
Dumbbell Hammer Curl: 3 hard sets	×	×	×

NOTES:

WORKOUT 4: UPPER BODY AND CORE			
EXERCISES	SETS		
Arnold Dumbbell Press: Warm-up and 3 hard sets	×	×	×
Close-Grip Bench Press: 3 hard sets	×	×	×
Dumbbell Side Lateral Raise: 3 hard sets	×	×	×
Seated Triceps Press: 3 hard sets	×	×	×
Crunch: 3 hard sets			

NOTES:

_____

_____

_____

WORKOUT 5: LOWER BODY (LEGS AND GLUTES)			
EXERCISES	SETS		
Barbell Front Squat: Warm-up and 3 hard sets	×	×	×
Leg Press: 3 hard sets	×	×	×
Romanian Deadlift: 3 hard sets	×	×	×
Hip Thrust: 3 hard sets	×	×	×

NOTES:

_____

_____

_____

5-DAY ROUTINE	PHASE 4	WEEK 35

WORKOUT 1: LOWER BODY (LEGS AND GLUTES)			
EXERCISES	SETS		
Barbell Squat: Warm-up and 3 hard sets	×	×	×
Dumbbell Lunge (Reverse): 3 hard sets	×	×	×
Leg Curl (Lying or Seated)*: 3 hard sets	×	×	×
Dumbbell Step-Up: 3 hard sets	×	×	×

NOTES:

WORKOUT 2: PUSH AND CORE			
EXERCISES	SETS		
Barbell Bench Press: Warm-up and 3 hard sets	×	×	×
Arnold Dumbbell Press: 3 hard sets	×	×	×
Dumbbell Bench Press: 3 hard sets	×	×	×
Dumbbell Rear Lateral Raise (Seated): 3 hard sets	×	×	×
Abdominal Rollout: 3 hard sets			

NOTES:

WORKOUT 3: PULL			
EXERCISES	SETS		
Barbell Deadlift: Warm-up and 3 hard sets	×	×	×
One-Arm Dumbbell Row: 3 hard sets	×	×	×
T-Bar Row: 3 hard sets	×	×	×
Dumbbell Hammer Curl: 3 hard sets	×	×	×

NOTES:

WORKOUT 4: UPPER BODY AND CORE			
EXERCISES	**SETS**		
Arnold Dumbbell Press: Warm-up and 3 hard sets	×	×	×
Close-Grip Bench Press: 3 hard sets	×	×	×
Dumbbell Side Lateral Raise: 3 hard sets	×	×	×
Seated Triceps Press: 3 hard sets	×	×	×
Crunch: 3 hard sets			

NOTES:

WORKOUT 5: LOWER BODY (LEGS AND GLUTES)			
EXERCISES	**SETS**		
Barbell Front Squat: Warm-up and 3 hard sets	×	×	×
Leg Press: 3 hard sets	×	×	×
Romanian Deadlift: 3 hard sets	×	×	×
Hip Thrust: 3 hard sets	×	×	×

NOTES:

5-DAY ROUTINE	DELOAD	WEEK 36

WORKOUT 1: DELOAD LEGS

EXERCISES	SETS		
Barbell Squat: Warm-up and 3 sets of 5 reps with last hard set weight	×	×	×
Romanian Deadlift: 3 sets of 5 reps with last hard set weight	×	×	×
Hip Thrust: 3 sets of 5 reps with last hard set weight	×	×	×

NOTES:

_____
_____

WORKOUT 2: DELOAD PUSH

EXERCISES	SETS		
Barbell Bench Press: Warm-up and 3 sets of 5 reps with last hard set weight	×	×	×
Seated Dumbbell Press: 3 sets of 5 reps with last hard set weight	×	×	×
Dumbbell Side Lateral Raise: 3 sets of 5 reps with last hard set weight	×	×	×

NOTES:

_____
_____

WORKOUT 3: DELOAD PULL

EXERCISES	SETS		
Barbell Deadlift: Warm-up and 3 sets of 5 reps with last hard set weight	×	×	×
Barbell Row: 3 sets of 5 reps with last hard set weight	×	×	×
Lat Pulldown (Wide-Grip): 3 sets of 5 reps with last hard set weight	×	×	×

NOTES:

_____
_____

4-DAY ROUTINE	PHASE 4	WEEK 28

WORKOUT 1: LOWER BODY (LEGS AND GLUTES)

EXERCISES	SETS		
Barbell Squat: Warm-up and 3 hard sets	×	×	×
Dumbbell Lunge (Reverse): 3 hard sets	×	×	×
Leg Curl (Lying or Seated)*: 3 hard sets	×	×	×
Dumbbell Step-Up: 3 hard sets	×	×	×

NOTES:

WORKOUT 2: UPPER BODY AND CORE

EXERCISES	SETS		
Barbell Bench Press: Warm-up and 3 hard sets	×	×	×
Arnold Dumbbell Press: 3 hard sets	×	×	×
Dumbbell Side Lateral Raise: 3 hard sets	×	×	×
Seated Triceps Press: 3 hard sets	×	×	×
Captain's Chair Leg Raise: 3 hard sets			

NOTES:

WORKOUT 3: PULL			
EXERCISES	**SETS**		
Barbell Deadlift: Warm-up and 3 hard sets	×	×	×
One-Arm Dumbbell Row: 3 hard sets	×	×	×
T-Bar Row: 3 hard sets	×	×	×
Dumbbell Hammer Curl: 3 hard sets	×	×	×

NOTES:

WORKOUT 4: LOWER BODY (LEGS AND GLUTES)			
EXERCISES	**SETS**		
Barbell Squat: Warm-up and 3 hard sets	×	×	×
Leg Press: 3 hard sets	×	×	×
Romanian Deadlift: 3 hard sets	×	×	×
Hip Thrust: 3 hard sets	×	×	×

NOTES:

| 4-DAY ROUTINE | PHASE 4 | WEEK 29 |

WORKOUT 1: LOWER BODY (LEGS AND GLUTES)			
EXERCISES	**SETS**		
Barbell Squat: Warm-up and 3 hard sets	×	×	×
Dumbbell Lunge (Reverse): 3 hard sets	×	×	×
Leg Curl (Lying or Seated)*: 3 hard sets	×	×	×
Dumbbell Step-Up: 3 hard sets	×	×	×

NOTES:

WORKOUT 2: UPPER BODY AND CORE			
EXERCISES	**SETS**		
Barbell Bench Press: Warm-up and 3 hard sets	×	×	×
Arnold Dumbbell Press: 3 hard sets	×	×	×
Dumbbell Side Lateral Raise: 3 hard sets	×	×	×
Seated Triceps Press: 3 hard sets	×	×	×
Captain's Chair Leg Raise: 3 hard sets			

NOTES:

WORKOUT 3: PULL			
EXERCISES	**SETS**		
Barbell Deadlift: Warm-up and 3 hard sets	✕	✕	✕
One-Arm Dumbbell Row: 3 hard sets	✕	✕	✕
T-Bar Row: 3 hard sets	✕	✕	✕
Dumbbell Hammer Curl: 3 hard sets	✕	✕	✕

NOTES:

_____

_____

_____

WORKOUT 4: LOWER BODY (LEGS AND GLUTES)			
EXERCISES	**SETS**		
Barbell Squat: Warm-up and 3 hard sets	✕	✕	✕
Leg Press: 3 hard sets	✕	✕	✕
Romanian Deadlift: 3 hard sets	✕	✕	✕
Hip Thrust: 3 hard sets	✕	✕	✕

NOTES:

_____

_____

_____

4-DAY ROUTINE	PHASE 4	WEEK 30

WORKOUT 1: LOWER BODY (LEGS AND GLUTES)			
EXERCISES	SETS		
Barbell Squat: Warm-up and 3 hard sets	×	×	×
Dumbbell Lunge (Reverse): 3 hard sets	×	×	×
Leg Curl (Lying or Seated)*: 3 hard sets	×	×	×
Dumbbell Step-Up: 3 hard sets	×	×	×

NOTES:

WORKOUT 2: UPPER BODY AND CORE			
EXERCISES	SETS		
Barbell Bench Press: Warm-up and 3 hard sets	×	×	×
Arnold Dumbbell Press: 3 hard sets	×	×	×
Dumbbell Side Lateral Raise: 3 hard sets	×	×	×
Seated Triceps Press: 3 hard sets	×	×	×
Captain's Chair Leg Raise: 3 hard sets			

NOTES:

WORKOUT 3: PULL			
EXERCISES	**SETS**		
Barbell Deadlift: Warm-up and 3 hard sets	×	×	×
One-Arm Dumbbell Row: 3 hard sets	×	×	×
T-Bar Row: 3 hard sets	×	×	×
Dumbbell Hammer Curl: 3 hard sets	×	×	×

NOTES:

WORKOUT 4: LOWER BODY (LEGS AND GLUTES)			
EXERCISES	**SETS**		
Barbell Squat: Warm-up and 3 hard sets	×	×	×
Leg Press: 3 hard sets	×	×	×
Romanian Deadlift: 3 hard sets	×	×	×
Hip Thrust: 3 hard sets	×	×	×

NOTES:

4-DAY ROUTINE | PHASE 4 | WEEK 31

WORKOUT 1: LOWER BODY (LEGS AND GLUTES)

EXERCISES	SETS		
Barbell Squat: Warm-up and 3 hard sets	×	×	×
Dumbbell Lunge (Reverse): 3 hard sets	×	×	×
Leg Curl (Lying or Seated)*: 3 hard sets	×	×	×
Dumbbell Step-Up: 3 hard sets	×	×	×

NOTES:

WORKOUT 2: UPPER BODY AND CORE

EXERCISES	SETS		
Barbell Bench Press: Warm-up and 3 hard sets	×	×	×
Arnold Dumbbell Press: 3 hard sets	×	×	×
Dumbbell Side Lateral Raise: 3 hard sets	×	×	×
Seated Triceps Press: 3 hard sets	×	×	×
Captain's Chair Leg Raise: 3 hard sets			

NOTES:

WORKOUT 3: PULL			
EXERCISES	**SETS**		
Barbell Deadlift: Warm-up and 3 hard sets	×	×	×
One-Arm Dumbbell Row: 3 hard sets	×	×	×
T-Bar Row: 3 hard sets	×	×	×
Dumbbell Hammer Curl: 3 hard sets	×	×	×

NOTES:

_____

_____

_____

WORKOUT 4: LOWER BODY (LEGS AND GLUTES)			
EXERCISES	**SETS**		
Barbell Squat: Warm-up and 3 hard sets	×	×	×
Leg Press: 3 hard sets	×	×	×
Romanian Deadlift: 3 hard sets	×	×	×
Hip Thrust: 3 hard sets	×	×	×

NOTES:

_____

_____

_____

| 4-DAY ROUTINE | PHASE 4 | WEEK 32 |

WORKOUT 1: LOWER BODY (LEGS AND GLUTES)

EXERCISES	SETS		
Barbell Squat: Warm-up and 3 hard sets	×	×	×
Dumbbell Lunge (Reverse): 3 hard sets	×	×	×
Leg Curl (Lying or Seated)*: 3 hard sets	×	×	×
Dumbbell Step-Up: 3 hard sets	×	×	×

NOTES:

WORKOUT 2: UPPER BODY AND CORE

EXERCISES	SETS		
Barbell Bench Press: Warm-up and 3 hard sets	×	×	×
Arnold Dumbbell Press: 3 hard sets	×	×	×
Dumbbell Side Lateral Raise: 3 hard sets	×	×	×
Seated Triceps Press: 3 hard sets	×	×	×
Captain's Chair Leg Raise: 3 hard sets			

NOTES:

WORKOUT 3: PULL			
EXERCISES	**SETS**		
Barbell Deadlift: Warm-up and 3 hard sets	×	×	×
One-Arm Dumbbell Row: 3 hard sets	×	×	×
T-Bar Row: 3 hard sets	×	×	×
Dumbbell Hammer Curl: 3 hard sets	×	×	×

NOTES:

_____

_____

_____

WORKOUT 4: LOWER BODY (LEGS AND GLUTES)			
EXERCISES	**SETS**		
Barbell Squat: Warm-up and 3 hard sets	×	×	×
Leg Press: 3 hard sets	×	×	×
Romanian Deadlift: 3 hard sets	×	×	×
Hip Thrust: 3 hard sets	×	×	×

NOTES:

_____

_____

_____

4-DAY ROUTINE	PHASE 4	WEEK 33

WORKOUT 1: LOWER BODY (LEGS AND GLUTES)

EXERCISES	SETS		
Barbell Squat: Warm-up and 3 hard sets	×	×	×
Dumbbell Lunge (Reverse): 3 hard sets	×	×	×
Leg Curl (Lying or Seated)*: 3 hard sets	×	×	×
Dumbbell Step-Up: 3 hard sets	×	×	×

NOTES:

WORKOUT 2: UPPER BODY AND CORE

EXERCISES	SETS		
Barbell Bench Press: Warm-up and 3 hard sets	×	×	×
Arnold Dumbbell Press: 3 hard sets	×	×	×
Dumbbell Side Lateral Raise: 3 hard sets	×	×	×
Seated Triceps Press: 3 hard sets	×	×	×
Captain's Chair Leg Raise: 3 hard sets			

NOTES:

WORKOUT 3: PULL			
EXERCISES	**SETS**		
Barbell Deadlift: Warm-up and 3 hard sets	×	×	×
One-Arm Dumbbell Row: 3 hard sets	×	×	×
T-Bar Row: 3 hard sets	×	×	×
Dumbbell Hammer Curl: 3 hard sets	×	×	×

NOTES:

_____

_____

_____

WORKOUT 4: LOWER BODY (LEGS AND GLUTES)			
EXERCISES	**SETS**		
Barbell Squat: Warm-up and 3 hard sets	×	×	×
Leg Press: 3 hard sets	×	×	×
Romanian Deadlift: 3 hard sets	×	×	×
Hip Thrust: 3 hard sets	×	×	×

NOTES:

_____

_____

_____

4-DAY ROUTINE	PHASE 4	WEEK 34

WORKOUT 1: LOWER BODY (LEGS AND GLUTES)

EXERCISES	SETS		
Barbell Squat: Warm-up and 3 hard sets	×	×	×
Dumbbell Lunge (Reverse): 3 hard sets	×	×	×
Leg Curl (Lying or Seated)*: 3 hard sets	×	×	×
Dumbbell Step-Up: 3 hard sets	×	×	×

NOTES:

WORKOUT 2: UPPER BODY AND CORE

EXERCISES	SETS		
Barbell Bench Press: Warm-up and 3 hard sets	×	×	×
Arnold Dumbbell Press: 3 hard sets	×	×	×
Dumbbell Side Lateral Raise: 3 hard sets	×	×	×
Seated Triceps Press: 3 hard sets	×	×	×
Captain's Chair Leg Raise: 3 hard sets			

NOTES:

WORKOUT 3: PULL			
EXERCISES	**SETS**		
Barbell Deadlift: Warm-up and 3 hard sets	×	×	×
One-Arm Dumbbell Row: 3 hard sets	×	×	×
T-Bar Row: 3 hard sets	×	×	×
Dumbbell Hammer Curl: 3 hard sets	×	×	×

NOTES:

WORKOUT 4: LOWER BODY (LEGS AND GLUTES)			
EXERCISES	**SETS**		
Barbell Squat: Warm-up and 3 hard sets	×	×	×
Leg Press: 3 hard sets	×	×	×
Romanian Deadlift: 3 hard sets	×	×	×
Hip Thrust: 3 hard sets	×	×	×

NOTES:

4-DAY ROUTINE	PHASE 4	WEEK 35

WORKOUT 1: LOWER BODY (LEGS AND GLUTES)

EXERCISES	SETS		
Barbell Squat: Warm-up and 3 hard sets	×	×	×
Dumbbell Lunge (Reverse): 3 hard sets	×	×	×
Leg Curl (Lying or Seated)*: 3 hard sets	×	×	×
Dumbbell Step-Up: 3 hard sets	×	×	×

NOTES:

WORKOUT 2: UPPER BODY AND CORE

EXERCISES	SETS		
Barbell Bench Press: Warm-up and 3 hard sets	×	×	×
Arnold Dumbbell Press: 3 hard sets	×	×	×
Dumbbell Side Lateral Raise: 3 hard sets	×	×	×
Seated Triceps Press: 3 hard sets	×	×	×
Captain's Chair Leg Raise: 3 hard sets			

NOTES:

WORKOUT 3: PULL			
EXERCISES	**SETS**		
Barbell Deadlift: Warm-up and 3 hard sets	×	×	×
One-Arm Dumbbell Row: 3 hard sets	×	×	×
T-Bar Row: 3 hard sets	×	×	×
Dumbbell Hammer Curl: 3 hard sets	×	×	×

NOTES:

_____

_____

_____

WORKOUT 4: LOWER BODY (LEGS AND GLUTES)			
EXERCISES	**SETS**		
Barbell Squat: Warm-up and 3 hard sets	×	×	×
Leg Press: 3 hard sets	×	×	×
Romanian Deadlift: 3 hard sets	×	×	×
Hip Thrust: 3 hard sets	×	×	×

NOTES:

_____

_____

_____

4-DAY ROUTINE	DELOAD	WEEK 36

WORKOUT 1: DELOAD LEGS

EXERCISES	SETS		
Barbell Squat: Warm-up and 3 sets of 5 reps with last hard set weight	×	×	×
Romanian Deadlift: 3 sets of 5 reps with last hard set weight	×	×	×
Hip Thrust: 3 sets of 5 reps with last hard set weight	×	×	×

NOTES:

WORKOUT 2: DELOAD PUSH

EXERCISES	SETS		
Barbell Bench Press: Warm-up and 3 sets of 5 reps with last hard set weight	×	×	×
Seated Dumbbell Press: 3 sets of 5 reps with last hard set weight	×	×	×
Dumbbell Bench Press: 3 sets of 5 reps with last hard set weight	×	×	×

NOTES:

WORKOUT 3: DELOAD PULL

EXERCISES	SETS		
Barbell Deadlift: Warm-up and 3 sets of 5 reps with last hard set weight	×	×	×
Barbell Row: 3 sets of 5 reps with last hard set weight	×	×	×
Lat Pulldown (Wide-Grip): 3 sets of 5 reps with last hard set weight	×	×	×

NOTES:

3-DAY ROUTINE	PHASE 4	WEEK 28

WORKOUT 1: LOWER BODY (LEGS AND GLUTES)

EXERCISES	SETS		
Barbell Squat: Warm-up and 3 hard sets	×	×	×
Dumbbell Lunge (Reverse): 3 hard sets	×	×	×
Leg Curl (Lying or Seated)*: 3 hard sets	×	×	×
Dumbbell Step-Up: 3 hard sets	×	×	×

NOTES:

WORKOUT 2: UPPER BODY AND CORE

EXERCISES	SETS		
Barbell Bench Press: Warm-up and 3 hard sets	×	×	×
Arnold Dumbbell Press: 3 hard sets	×	×	×
Dumbbell Rear Lateral Raise (Seated): 3 hard sets	×	×	×
Seated Triceps Press: 3 hard sets	×	×	×
Abdominal Rollout: 3 hard sets			

NOTES:

WORKOUT 3: LOWER BODY AND PULL (LEGS AND BACK)

EXERCISES	SETS		
Barbell Squat: Warm-up and 3 hard sets	×	×	×
Barbell Deadlift: Warm-up and 3 hard sets	×	×	×
Lat Pulldown (Close-Grip): 3 hard sets	×	×	×
Seated Cable Row (Close-Grip): 3 hard sets	×	×	×
Barbell Curl: 3 hard sets	×	×	×

NOTES:

| 3-DAY ROUTINE | PHASE 4 | WEEK 29 |

WORKOUT 1: LOWER BODY (LEGS AND GLUTES)

EXERCISES	SETS		
Barbell Squat: Warm-up and 3 hard sets	×	×	×
Dumbbell Lunge (Reverse): 3 hard sets	×	×	×
Leg Curl (Lying or Seated)*: 3 hard sets	×	×	×
Dumbbell Step-Up: 3 hard sets	×	×	×

NOTES:

WORKOUT 2: UPPER BODY AND CORE

EXERCISES	SETS		
Barbell Bench Press: Warm-up and 3 hard sets	×	×	×
Arnold Dumbbell Press: 3 hard sets	×	×	×
Dumbbell Rear Lateral Raise (Seated): 3 hard sets	×	×	×
Seated Triceps Press: 3 hard sets	×	×	×
Abdominal Rollout: 3 hard sets			

NOTES:

WORKOUT 3: LOWER BODY AND PULL (LEGS AND BACK)

EXERCISES	SETS		
Barbell Squat: Warm-up and 3 hard sets	×	×	×
Barbell Deadlift: Warm-up and 3 hard sets	×	×	×
Lat Pulldown (Close-Grip): 3 hard sets	×	×	×
Seated Cable Row (Close-Grip): 3 hard sets	×	×	×
Barbell Curl: 3 hard sets	×	×	×

NOTES:

| 3-DAY ROUTINE | PHASE 4 | WEEK 30 |

WORKOUT 1: LOWER BODY (LEGS AND GLUTES)

EXERCISES	SETS		
Barbell Squat: Warm-up and 3 hard sets	×	×	×
Dumbbell Lunge (Reverse): 3 hard sets	×	×	×
Leg Curl (Lying or Seated)*: 3 hard sets	×	×	×
Dumbbell Step-Up: 3 hard sets	×	×	×

NOTES:

WORKOUT 2: UPPER BODY AND CORE

EXERCISES	SETS		
Barbell Bench Press: Warm-up and 3 hard sets	×	×	×
Arnold Dumbbell Press: 3 hard sets	×	×	×
Dumbbell Rear Lateral Raise (Seated): 3 hard sets	×	×	×
Seated Triceps Press: 3 hard sets	×	×	×
Abdominal Rollout: 3 hard sets			

NOTES:

WORKOUT 3: LOWER BODY AND PULL (LEGS AND BACK)

EXERCISES	SETS		
Barbell Squat: Warm-up and 3 hard sets	×	×	×
Barbell Deadlift: Warm-up and 3 hard sets	×	×	×
Lat Pulldown (Close-Grip): 3 hard sets	×	×	×
Seated Cable Row (Close-Grip): 3 hard sets	×	×	×
Barbell Curl: 3 hard sets	×	×	×

NOTES:

3-DAY ROUTINE	PHASE 4	WEEK 31

WORKOUT 1: LOWER BODY (LEGS AND GLUTES)			
EXERCISES	SETS		
Barbell Squat: Warm-up and 3 hard sets	×	×	×
Dumbbell Lunge (Reverse): 3 hard sets	×	×	×
Leg Curl (Lying or Seated)*: 3 hard sets	×	×	×
Dumbbell Step-Up: 3 hard sets	×	×	×

NOTES:

WORKOUT 2: UPPER BODY AND CORE			
EXERCISES	SETS		
Barbell Bench Press: Warm-up and 3 hard sets	×	×	×
Arnold Dumbbell Press: 3 hard sets	×	×	×
Dumbbell Rear Lateral Raise (Seated): 3 hard sets	×	×	×
Seated Triceps Press: 3 hard sets	×	×	×
Abdominal Rollout: 3 hard sets			

NOTES:

WORKOUT 3: LOWER BODY AND PULL (LEGS AND BACK)			
EXERCISES	SETS		
Barbell Squat: Warm-up and 3 hard sets	×	×	×
Barbell Deadlift: Warm-up and 3 hard sets	×	×	×
Lat Pulldown (Close-Grip): 3 hard sets	×	×	×
Seated Cable Row (Close-Grip): 3 hard sets	×	×	×
Barbell Curl: 3 hard sets	×	×	×

NOTES:

3-DAY ROUTINE	PHASE 4	WEEK 32

WORKOUT 1: LOWER BODY (LEGS AND GLUTES)			
EXERCISES	SETS		
Barbell Squat: Warm-up and 3 hard sets	×	×	×
Dumbbell Lunge (Reverse): 3 hard sets	×	×	×
Leg Curl (Lying or Seated)*: 3 hard sets	×	×	×
Dumbbell Step-Up: 3 hard sets	×	×	×

NOTES:

WORKOUT 2: UPPER BODY AND CORE			
EXERCISES	SETS		
Barbell Bench Press: Warm-up and 3 hard sets	×	×	×
Arnold Dumbbell Press: 3 hard sets	×	×	×
Dumbbell Rear Lateral Raise (Seated): 3 hard sets	×	×	×
Seated Triceps Press: 3 hard sets	×	×	×
Abdominal Rollout: 3 hard sets			

NOTES:

WORKOUT 3: LOWER BODY AND PULL (LEGS AND BACK)			
EXERCISES	SETS		
Barbell Squat: Warm-up and 3 hard sets	×	×	×
Barbell Deadlift: Warm-up and 3 hard sets	×	×	×
Lat Pulldown (Close-Grip): 3 hard sets	×	×	×
Seated Cable Row (Close-Grip): 3 hard sets	×	×	×
Barbell Curl: 3 hard sets	×	×	×

NOTES:

3-DAY ROUTINE	PHASE 4	WEEK 33

WORKOUT 1: LOWER BODY (LEGS AND GLUTES)

EXERCISES	SETS		
Barbell Squat: Warm-up and 3 hard sets	×	×	×
Dumbbell Lunge (Reverse): 3 hard sets	×	×	×
Leg Curl (Lying or Seated)*: 3 hard sets	×	×	×
Dumbbell Step-Up: 3 hard sets	×	×	×

NOTES:

WORKOUT 2: UPPER BODY AND CORE

EXERCISES	SETS		
Barbell Bench Press: Warm-up and 3 hard sets	×	×	×
Arnold Dumbbell Press: 3 hard sets	×	×	×
Dumbbell Rear Lateral Raise (Seated): 3 hard sets	×	×	×
Seated Triceps Press: 3 hard sets	×	×	×
Abdominal Rollout: 3 hard sets			

NOTES:

WORKOUT 3: LOWER BODY AND PULL (LEGS AND BACK)

EXERCISES	SETS		
Barbell Squat: Warm-up and 3 hard sets	×	×	×
Barbell Deadlift: Warm-up and 3 hard sets	×	×	×
Lat Pulldown (Close-Grip): 3 hard sets	×	×	×
Seated Cable Row (Close-Grip): 3 hard sets	×	×	×
Barbell Curl: 3 hard sets	×	×	×

NOTES:

3-DAY ROUTINE	PHASE 4	WEEK 34

WORKOUT 1: LOWER BODY (LEGS AND GLUTES)			
EXERCISES	SETS		
Barbell Squat: Warm-up and 3 hard sets	×	×	×
Dumbbell Lunge (Reverse): 3 hard sets	×	×	×
Leg Curl (Lying or Seated)*: 3 hard sets	×	×	×
Dumbbell Step-Up: 3 hard sets	×	×	×

NOTES:

WORKOUT 2: UPPER BODY AND CORE			
EXERCISES	SETS		
Barbell Bench Press: Warm-up and 3 hard sets	×	×	×
Arnold Dumbbell Press: 3 hard sets	×	×	×
Dumbbell Rear Lateral Raise (Seated): 3 hard sets	×	×	×
Seated Triceps Press: 3 hard sets	×	×	×
Abdominal Rollout: 3 hard sets			

NOTES:

WORKOUT 3: LOWER BODY AND PULL (LEGS AND BACK)			
EXERCISES	SETS		
Barbell Squat: Warm-up and 3 hard sets	×	×	×
Barbell Deadlift: Warm-up and 3 hard sets	×	×	×
Lat Pulldown (Close-Grip): 3 hard sets	×	×	×
Seated Cable Row (Close-Grip): 3 hard sets	×	×	×
Barbell Curl: 3 hard sets	×	×	×

NOTES:

3-DAY ROUTINE	PHASE 4	WEEK 35

WORKOUT 1: LOWER BODY (LEGS AND GLUTES)

EXERCISES	SETS		
Barbell Squat: Warm-up and 3 hard sets	×	×	×
Dumbbell Lunge (Reverse): 3 hard sets	×	×	×
Leg Curl (Lying or Seated)*: 3 hard sets	×	×	×
Dumbbell Step-Up: 3 hard sets	×	×	×

NOTES:

WORKOUT 2: UPPER BODY AND CORE

EXERCISES	SETS		
Barbell Bench Press: Warm-up and 3 hard sets	×	×	×
Arnold Dumbbell Press: 3 hard sets	×	×	×
Dumbbell Rear Lateral Raise (Seated): 3 hard sets	×	×	×
Seated Triceps Press: 3 hard sets	×	×	×
Abdominal Rollout: 3 hard sets			

NOTES:

WORKOUT 3: LOWER BODY AND PULL (LEGS AND BACK)

EXERCISES	SETS		
Barbell Squat: Warm-up and 3 hard sets	×	×	×
Barbell Deadlift: Warm-up and 3 hard sets	×	×	×
Lat Pulldown (Close-Grip): 3 hard sets	×	×	×
Seated Cable Row (Close-Grip): 3 hard sets	×	×	×
Barbell Curl: 3 hard sets	×	×	×

NOTES:

3-DAY ROUTINE	DELOAD	WEEK 36

WORKOUT 1: DELOAD LEGS

EXERCISES	SETS		
Barbell Squat: Warm-up and 3 sets of 5 reps with last hard set weight	×	×	×
Romanian Deadlift: 3 sets of 5 reps with last hard set weight	×	×	×
Hip Thrust: 3 sets of 5 reps with last hard set weight	×	×	×

NOTES:

WORKOUT 2: DELOAD PUSH

EXERCISES	SETS		
Barbell Bench Press: Warm-up and 3 sets of 5 reps with last hard set weight	×	×	×
Seated Dumbbell Press: 3 sets of 5 reps with last hard set weight	×	×	×
Dumbbell Bench Press: 3 sets of 5 reps with last hard set weight	×	×	×

NOTES:

WORKOUT 3: DELOAD PULL

EXERCISES	SETS		
Barbell Deadlift: Warm-up and 3 sets of 5 reps with last hard set weight	×	×	×
Barbell Row: 3 sets of 5 reps with last hard set weight	×	×	×
Lat Pulldown (Wide-Grip): 3 sets of 5 reps with last hard set weight	×	×	×

NOTES:

Look at you! On a roll!

As the meatheads say, there are no brakes on this gains train.

Seriously, though, hats off—you're doing great work.

Many people can't stick to anything for more than six months, much less a challenging diet and exercise plan. Yet here you are.

Furthermore, here you are staying the course despite the speed bumps that you've undoubtedly hit along the way—low-energy days, scheduling kerfuffles, sickness, sleepless nights—in other words, the "fuckery" of life, as I like to call it.

You didn't let any of that stop you, which proves beyond a shadow of a doubt that you're in it to win it and have what it takes.

As always, let's get some new measurements and pictures before moving ahead.

First, take the following body measurements first thing in the morning, nude, after using the bathroom and before eating or drinking anything:

1. Weight

2. Waist circumference

3. OPTIONAL: Hip circumference

4. OPTIONAL: Upper-leg circumference

5. OPTIONAL: Flexed arms

Then, take flexed and unflexed pictures from the front, back, and sides, and store them in an album or folder that you can easily locate later.

Remember to show as much skin as you feel comfortable with. The more the better because it will give you the best idea of how your body is responding to the program.

Keep up the good work!

I'D RATHER REGRET THE THINGS I'VE DONE THAN REGRET THE THINGS I HAVEN'T DONE.

—LUCILLE BALL

THINNER LEANER STRONGER PHASE 5

I know you don't need any congratulations at this point, but I want to give you a high five anyway because you've invested a lot of time and sweat into this journey, and I'm proud of you.

No matter how much you may be enjoying your workouts, you've probably noticed that it has gotten much more difficult to increase the weight on your exercises. This is very normal. Most people can progress like clockwork for the first six to nine months, but then the game changes and improvements are harder to come by.

The primary reason for this is that your body is hyper-responsive to weightlifting when you first start, so you're able to move ahead in leaps and bounds. In time, though, this responsiveness declines and thus progress slows.

The fitness game is like anything else. The better you get at it, the harder it is to continue getting better.

Don't be discouraged by this, though. You have all the tools you need to not only continue progressing in your training, but to ultimately get the body you really want. You just have to keep using them.

So, on the following pages, you'll find your next eight weeks of hard training and deload. As before, choose the split that best suits your goals and circumstances, and stick with it until you've completed this fifth phase.

As usual, let's reflect on the last phase before moving on.

Answer the following questions, and if you have a lot to say, jot it down so you can easily refer back to it.

→ What are three things in your diet and/or training that went particularly well in the last phase? Why?

→ What's one thing you could have done better? Why?

→ What's one thing you can do to make your next phase even better than the last?

Have fun and I'll see you on the other end of this next sprint!

5-DAY ROUTINE	PHASE 5	WEEK 37

WORKOUT 1: LOWER BODY (LEGS AND GLUTES)

EXERCISES	SETS		
Barbell Squat: Warm-up and 3 hard sets	×	×	×
Barbell Single-Leg Split Squat : 3 hard sets	×	×	×
Romanian Deadlift: 3 hard sets	×	×	×
Hip Thrust: 3 hard sets	×	×	×

NOTES:

WORKOUT 2: PUSH AND CORE

EXERCISES	SETS		
Barbell Bench Press: Warm-up and 3 hard sets	×	×	×
Dumbbell Bench Press: 3 hard sets	×	×	×
Dip: 3 hard sets	×	×	×
Dumbbell Side Lateral Raise: 3 hard sets	×	×	×
Hanging Leg Raise: 3 hard sets			

NOTES:

WORKOUT 3: PULL

EXERCISES	SETS		
Barbell Deadlift: Warm-up and 3 hard sets	×	×	×
Barbell Row: 3 hard sets	×	×	×
Seated Cable Row (Close-Grip): 3 hard sets	×	×	×
E-Z Bar Curl: 3 hard sets	×	×	×

NOTES:

WORKOUT 4: UPPER BODY AND CORE			
EXERCISES	**SETS**		
Seated Dumbbell Press: Warm-up and 3 hard sets	×	×	×
Dumbbell Bench Press: 3 hard sets	×	×	×
Barbell Rear Delt Row: 3 hard sets	×	×	×
Lying Triceps Extension: 3 hard sets	×	×	×
Weighted Sit-Up: 3 hard sets	×	×	×

NOTES:

_____

_____

_____

WORKOUT 5: LOWER BODY (LEGS AND GLUTES)			
EXERCISES	**SETS**		
Barbell Squat: Warm-up and 3 hard sets	×	×	×
Barbell Lunge (In-Place): 3 hard sets	×	×	×
Leg Curl (Lying or Seated)*: 3 hard sets	×	×	×
Glute Blaster: 3 hard sets	×	×	×

NOTES:

_____

_____

_____

5-DAY ROUTINE	PHASE 5	WEEK 38

WORKOUT 1: LOWER BODY (LEGS AND GLUTES)			
EXERCISES	SETS		
Barbell Squat: Warm-up and 3 hard sets	×	×	×
Barbell Single-Leg Split Squat : 3 hard sets	×	×	×
Romanian Deadlift: 3 hard sets	×	×	×
Hip Thrust: 3 hard sets	×	×	×

NOTES:

WORKOUT 2: PUSH AND CORE			
EXERCISES	SETS		
Barbell Bench Press: Warm-up and 3 hard sets	×	×	×
Dumbbell Bench Press: 3 hard sets	×	×	×
Dip: 3 hard sets	×	×	×
Dumbbell Side Lateral Raise: 3 hard sets	×	×	×
Hanging Leg Raise: 3 hard sets			

NOTES:

WORKOUT 3: PULL			
EXERCISES	SETS		
Barbell Deadlift: Warm-up and 3 hard sets	×	×	×
Barbell Row: 3 hard sets	×	×	×
Seated Cable Row (Close-Grip): 3 hard sets	×	×	×
E-Z Bar Curl: 3 hard sets	×	×	×

NOTES:

WORKOUT 4: UPPER BODY AND CORE			
EXERCISES	**SETS**		
Seated Dumbbell Press: Warm-up and 3 hard sets	×	×	×
Dumbbell Bench Press: 3 hard sets	×	×	×
Barbell Rear Delt Row: 3 hard sets	×	×	×
Lying Triceps Extension: 3 hard sets	×	×	×
Weighted Sit-Up: 3 hard sets	×	×	×

NOTES:

WORKOUT 5: LOWER BODY (LEGS AND GLUTES)			
EXERCISES	**SETS**		
Barbell Squat: Warm-up and 3 hard sets	×	×	×
Barbell Lunge (In-Place): 3 hard sets	×	×	×
Leg Curl (Lying or Seated)*: 3 hard sets	×	×	×
Glute Blaster: 3 hard sets	×	×	×

NOTES:

5-DAY ROUTINE	PHASE 5	WEEK 39

WORKOUT 1: LOWER BODY (LEGS AND GLUTES)			
EXERCISES	**SETS**		
Barbell Squat: Warm-up and 3 hard sets	×	×	×
Barbell Single-Leg Split Squat : 3 hard sets	×	×	×
Romanian Deadlift: 3 hard sets	×	×	×
Hip Thrust: 3 hard sets	×	×	×

NOTES:

WORKOUT 2: PUSH AND CORE			
EXERCISES	**SETS**		
Barbell Bench Press: Warm-up and 3 hard sets	×	×	×
Dumbbell Bench Press: 3 hard sets	×	×	×
Dip: 3 hard sets	×	×	×
Dumbbell Side Lateral Raise: 3 hard sets	×	×	×
Hanging Leg Raise: 3 hard sets			

NOTES:

WORKOUT 3: PULL			
EXERCISES	**SETS**		
Barbell Deadlift: Warm-up and 3 hard sets	×	×	×
Barbell Row: 3 hard sets	×	×	×
Seated Cable Row (Close-Grip): 3 hard sets	×	×	×
E-Z Bar Curl: 3 hard sets	×	×	×

NOTES:

WORKOUT 4: UPPER BODY AND CORE			
EXERCISES	**SETS**		
Seated Dumbbell Press: Warm-up and 3 hard sets	×	×	×
Dumbbell Bench Press: 3 hard sets	×	×	×
Barbell Rear Delt Row: 3 hard sets	×	×	×
Lying Triceps Extension: 3 hard sets	×	×	×
Weighted Sit-Up: 3 hard sets	×	×	×

NOTES:

_____

_____

WORKOUT 5: LOWER BODY (LEGS AND GLUTES)			
EXERCISES	**SETS**		
Barbell Squat: Warm-up and 3 hard sets	×	×	×
Barbell Lunge (In-Place): 3 hard sets	×	×	×
Leg Curl (Lying or Seated)*: 3 hard sets	×	×	×
Glute Blaster: 3 hard sets	×	×	×

NOTES:

_____

_____

5-DAY ROUTINE — PHASE 5 — WEEK 40

WORKOUT 1: LOWER BODY (LEGS AND GLUTES)

EXERCISES	SETS		
Barbell Squat: Warm-up and 3 hard sets	×	×	×
Barbell Single-Leg Split Squat : 3 hard sets	×	×	×
Romanian Deadlift: 3 hard sets	×	×	×
Hip Thrust: 3 hard sets	×	×	×

NOTES:

WORKOUT 2: PUSH AND CORE

EXERCISES	SETS		
Barbell Bench Press: Warm-up and 3 hard sets	×	×	×
Dumbbell Bench Press: 3 hard sets	×	×	×
Dip: 3 hard sets	×	×	×
Dumbbell Side Lateral Raise: 3 hard sets	×	×	×
Hanging Leg Raise: 3 hard sets			

NOTES:

WORKOUT 3: PULL

EXERCISES	SETS		
Barbell Deadlift: Warm-up and 3 hard sets	×	×	×
Barbell Row: 3 hard sets	×	×	×
Seated Cable Row (Close-Grip): 3 hard sets	×	×	×
E-Z Bar Curl: 3 hard sets	×	×	×

NOTES:

WORKOUT 4: UPPER BODY AND CORE			
EXERCISES	**SETS**		
Seated Dumbbell Press: Warm-up and 3 hard sets	×	×	×
Dumbbell Bench Press: 3 hard sets	×	×	×
Barbell Rear Delt Row: 3 hard sets	×	×	×
Lying Triceps Extension: 3 hard sets	×	×	×
Weighted Sit-Up: 3 hard sets	×	×	×

NOTES:

WORKOUT 5: LOWER BODY (LEGS AND GLUTES)			
EXERCISES	**SETS**		
Barbell Squat: Warm-up and 3 hard sets	×	×	×
Barbell Lunge (In-Place): 3 hard sets	×	×	×
Leg Curl (Lying or Seated)*: 3 hard sets	×	×	×
Glute Blaster: 3 hard sets	×	×	×

NOTES:

| 5-DAY ROUTINE | PHASE 5 | WEEK 41 |

WORKOUT 1: LOWER BODY (LEGS AND GLUTES)

EXERCISES	SETS		
Barbell Squat: Warm-up and 3 hard sets	×	×	×
Barbell Single-Leg Split Squat : 3 hard sets	×	×	×
Romanian Deadlift: 3 hard sets	×	×	×
Hip Thrust: 3 hard sets	×	×	×

NOTES:

WORKOUT 2: PUSH AND CORE

EXERCISES	SETS		
Barbell Bench Press: Warm-up and 3 hard sets	×	×	×
Dumbbell Bench Press: 3 hard sets	×	×	×
Dip: 3 hard sets	×	×	×
Dumbbell Side Lateral Raise: 3 hard sets	×	×	×
Hanging Leg Raise: 3 hard sets			

NOTES:

WORKOUT 3: PULL

EXERCISES	SETS		
Barbell Deadlift: Warm-up and 3 hard sets	×	×	×
Barbell Row: 3 hard sets	×	×	×
Seated Cable Row (Close-Grip): 3 hard sets	×	×	×
E-Z Bar Curl: 3 hard sets	×	×	×

NOTES:

WORKOUT 4: UPPER BODY AND CORE			
EXERCISES	**SETS**		
Seated Dumbbell Press: Warm-up and 3 hard sets	×	×	×
Dumbbell Bench Press: 3 hard sets	×	×	×
Barbell Rear Delt Row: 3 hard sets	×	×	×
Lying Triceps Extension: 3 hard sets	×	×	×
Weighted Sit-Up: 3 hard sets	×	×	×

NOTES:

_____

_____

_____

WORKOUT 5: LOWER BODY (LEGS AND GLUTES)			
EXERCISES	**SETS**		
Barbell Squat: Warm-up and 3 hard sets	×	×	×
Barbell Lunge (In-Place): 3 hard sets	×	×	×
Leg Curl (Lying or Seated)*: 3 hard sets	×	×	×
Glute Blaster: 3 hard sets	×	×	×

NOTES:

_____

_____

_____

5-DAY ROUTINE	PHASE 5	WEEK 42

WORKOUT 1: LOWER BODY (LEGS AND GLUTES)			
EXERCISES	**SETS**		
Barbell Squat: Warm-up and 3 hard sets	×	×	×
Barbell Single-Leg Split Squat : 3 hard sets	×	×	×
Romanian Deadlift: 3 hard sets	×	×	×
Hip Thrust: 3 hard sets	×	×	×

NOTES:

WORKOUT 2: PUSH AND CORE			
EXERCISES	**SETS**		
Barbell Bench Press: Warm-up and 3 hard sets	×	×	×
Dumbbell Bench Press: 3 hard sets	×	×	×
Dip: 3 hard sets	×	×	×
Dumbbell Side Lateral Raise: 3 hard sets	×	×	×
Hanging Leg Raise: 3 hard sets			

NOTES:

WORKOUT 3: PULL			
EXERCISES	**SETS**		
Barbell Deadlift: Warm-up and 3 hard sets	×	×	×
Barbell Row: 3 hard sets	×	×	×
Seated Cable Row (Close-Grip): 3 hard sets	×	×	×
E-Z Bar Curl: 3 hard sets	×	×	×

NOTES:

WORKOUT 4: UPPER BODY AND CORE			
EXERCISES	**SETS**		
Seated Dumbbell Press: Warm-up and 3 hard sets	×	×	×
Dumbbell Bench Press: 3 hard sets	×	×	×
Barbell Rear Delt Row: 3 hard sets	×	×	×
Lying Triceps Extension: 3 hard sets	×	×	×
Weighted Sit-Up: 3 hard sets	×	×	×

NOTES:

WORKOUT 5: LOWER BODY (LEGS AND GLUTES)			
EXERCISES	**SETS**		
Barbell Squat: Warm-up and 3 hard sets	×	×	×
Barbell Lunge (In-Place): 3 hard sets	×	×	×
Leg Curl (Lying or Seated)*: 3 hard sets	×	×	×
Glute Blaster: 3 hard sets	×	×	×

NOTES:

5-DAY ROUTINE	PHASE 5	WEEK 43

WORKOUT 1: LOWER BODY (LEGS AND GLUTES)

EXERCISES	SETS		
Barbell Squat: Warm-up and 3 hard sets	×	×	×
Barbell Single-Leg Split Squat : 3 hard sets	×	×	×
Romanian Deadlift: 3 hard sets	×	×	×
Hip Thrust: 3 hard sets	×	×	×

NOTES:

WORKOUT 2: PUSH AND CORE

EXERCISES	SETS		
Barbell Bench Press: Warm-up and 3 hard sets	×	×	×
Dumbbell Bench Press: 3 hard sets	×	×	×
Dip: 3 hard sets	×	×	×
Dumbbell Side Lateral Raise: 3 hard sets	×	×	×
Hanging Leg Raise: 3 hard sets			

NOTES:

WORKOUT 3: PULL

EXERCISES	SETS		
Barbell Deadlift: Warm-up and 3 hard sets	×	×	×
Barbell Row: 3 hard sets	×	×	×
Seated Cable Row (Close-Grip): 3 hard sets	×	×	×
E-Z Bar Curl: 3 hard sets	×	×	×

NOTES:

WORKOUT 4: UPPER BODY AND CORE			
EXERCISES	**SETS**		
Seated Dumbbell Press: Warm-up and 3 hard sets	×	×	×
Dumbbell Bench Press: 3 hard sets	×	×	×
Barbell Rear Delt Row: 3 hard sets	×	×	×
Lying Triceps Extension: 3 hard sets	×	×	×
Weighted Sit-Up: 3 hard sets	×	×	×

NOTES:

_____

_____

_____

WORKOUT 5: LOWER BODY (LEGS AND GLUTES)			
EXERCISES	**SETS**		
Barbell Squat: Warm-up and 3 hard sets	×	×	×
Barbell Lunge (In-Place): 3 hard sets	×	×	×
Leg Curl (Lying or Seated)*: 3 hard sets	×	×	×
Glute Blaster: 3 hard sets	×	×	×

NOTES:

_____

_____

_____

5-DAY ROUTINE	PHASE 5	WEEK 44

WORKOUT 1: LOWER BODY (LEGS AND GLUTES)

EXERCISES	SETS		
Barbell Squat: Warm-up and 3 hard sets	×	×	×
Barbell Single-Leg Split Squat : 3 hard sets	×	×	×
Romanian Deadlift: 3 hard sets	×	×	×
Hip Thrust: 3 hard sets	×	×	×

NOTES:

WORKOUT 2: PUSH AND CORE

EXERCISES	SETS		
Barbell Bench Press: Warm-up and 3 hard sets	×	×	×
Dumbbell Bench Press: 3 hard sets	×	×	×
Dip: 3 hard sets	×	×	×
Dumbbell Side Lateral Raise: 3 hard sets	×	×	×
Hanging Leg Raise: 3 hard sets			

NOTES:

WORKOUT 3: PULL

EXERCISES	SETS		
Barbell Deadlift: Warm-up and 3 hard sets	×	×	×
Barbell Row: 3 hard sets	×	×	×
Seated Cable Row (Close-Grip): 3 hard sets	×	×	×
E-Z Bar Curl: 3 hard sets	×	×	×

NOTES:

WORKOUT 4: UPPER BODY AND CORE			
EXERCISES	**SETS**		
Seated Dumbbell Press: Warm-up and 3 hard sets	✕	✕	✕
Dumbbell Bench Press: 3 hard sets	✕	✕	✕
Barbell Rear Delt Row: 3 hard sets	✕	✕	✕
Lying Triceps Extension: 3 hard sets	✕	✕	✕
Weighted Sit-Up: 3 hard sets	✕	✕	✕

NOTES:

WORKOUT 5: LOWER BODY (LEGS AND GLUTES)			
EXERCISES	**SETS**		
Barbell Squat: Warm-up and 3 hard sets	✕	✕	✕
Barbell Lunge (In-Place): 3 hard sets	✕	✕	✕
Leg Curl (Lying or Seated)*: 3 hard sets	✕	✕	✕
Glute Blaster: 3 hard sets	✕	✕	✕

NOTES:

5-DAY ROUTINE	DELOAD	WEEK 45

WORKOUT 1: DELOAD LEGS

EXERCISES	SETS		
Barbell Squat: Warm-up and 3 sets of 5 reps with last hard set weight	×	×	×
Romanian Deadlift: 3 sets of 5 reps with last hard set weight	×	×	×
Hip Thrust: 3 sets of 5 reps with last hard set weight	×	×	×

NOTES:

_____

_____

_____

WORKOUT 2: DELOAD PUSH

EXERCISES	SETS		
Barbell Bench Press: Warm-up and 3 sets of 5 reps with last hard set weight	×	×	×
Seated Dumbbell Press: 3 sets of 5 reps with last hard set weight	×	×	×
Dumbbell Side Lateral Raise: 3 sets of 5 reps with last hard set weight	×	×	×

NOTES:

_____

_____

_____

WORKOUT 3: DELOAD PULL

EXERCISES	SETS		
Barbell Deadlift: Warm-up and 3 sets of 5 reps with last hard set weight	×	×	×
Barbell Row: 3 sets of 5 reps with last hard set weight	×	×	×
Lat Pulldown (Wide-Grip): 3 sets of 5 reps with last hard set weight	×	×	×

NOTES:

_____

_____

_____

4-DAY ROUTINE	PHASE 5	WEEK 37

WORKOUT 1: LOWER BODY (LEGS AND GLUTES)

EXERCISES	SETS		
Barbell Squat: Warm-up and 3 hard sets	×	×	×
Barbell Single-Leg Split Squat : 3 hard sets	×	×	×
Romanian Deadlift: 3 hard sets	×	×	×
Hip Thrust: 3 hard sets	×	×	×

NOTES:

_____

_____

_____

WORKOUT 2: UPPER BODY AND CORE

EXERCISES	SETS		
Barbell Bench Press: Warm-up and 3 hard sets	×	×	×
Dip: 3 hard sets	×	×	×
Barbell Rear Delt Row: 3 hard sets	×	×	×
Lying Triceps Extension: 3 hard sets	×	×	×
Weighted Sit-Up : 3 hard sets	×	×	×

NOTES:

_____

_____

_____

WORKOUT 3: PULL			
EXERCISES	**SETS**		
Barbell Deadlift: Warm-up and 3 hard sets	×	×	×
Barbell Row: 3 hard sets	×	×	×
Seated Cable Row (Close-Grip): 3 hard sets	×	×	×
E-Z Bar Curl: 3 hard sets	×	×	×

NOTES:

_____

_____

_____

WORKOUT 4: LOWER BODY (LEGS AND GLUTES)			
EXERCISES	**SETS**		
Barbell Squat: Warm-up and 3 hard sets	×	×	×
Barbell Lunge (In-Place): 3 hard sets	×	×	×
Leg Curl (Lying or Seated)*: 3 hard sets	×	×	×
Glute Blaster: 3 hard sets	×	×	×

NOTES:

_____

_____

_____

4-DAY ROUTINE	PHASE 5	WEEK 38

WORKOUT 1: LOWER BODY (LEGS AND GLUTES)

EXERCISES	SETS		
Barbell Squat: Warm-up and 3 hard sets	×	×	×
Barbell Single-Leg Split Squat : 3 hard sets	×	×	×
Romanian Deadlift: 3 hard sets	×	×	×
Hip Thrust: 3 hard sets	×	×	×

NOTES:

WORKOUT 2: UPPER BODY AND CORE

EXERCISES	SETS		
Barbell Bench Press: Warm-up and 3 hard sets	×	×	×
Dip: 3 hard sets	×	×	×
Barbell Rear Delt Row: 3 hard sets	×	×	×
Lying Triceps Extension: 3 hard sets	×	×	×
Weighted Sit-Up : 3 hard sets	×	×	×

NOTES:

WORKOUT 3: PULL			
EXERCISES	**SETS**		
Barbell Deadlift: Warm-up and 3 hard sets	×	×	×
Barbell Row: 3 hard sets	×	×	×
Seated Cable Row (Close-Grip): 3 hard sets	×	×	×
E-Z Bar Curl: 3 hard sets	×	×	×

NOTES:

WORKOUT 4: LOWER BODY (LEGS AND GLUTES)			
EXERCISES	**SETS**		
Barbell Squat: Warm-up and 3 hard sets	×	×	×
Barbell Lunge (In-Place): 3 hard sets	×	×	×
Leg Curl (Lying or Seated)*: 3 hard sets	×	×	×
Glute Blaster: 3 hard sets	×	×	×

NOTES:

4-DAY ROUTINE	PHASE 5	WEEK 39

WORKOUT 1: LOWER BODY (LEGS AND GLUTES)

EXERCISES	SETS		
Barbell Squat: Warm-up and 3 hard sets	×	×	×
Barbell Single-Leg Split Squat : 3 hard sets	×	×	×
Romanian Deadlift: 3 hard sets	×	×	×
Hip Thrust: 3 hard sets	×	×	×

NOTES:

WORKOUT 2: UPPER BODY AND CORE

EXERCISES	SETS		
Barbell Bench Press: Warm-up and 3 hard sets	×	×	×
Dip: 3 hard sets	×	×	×
Barbell Rear Delt Row: 3 hard sets	×	×	×
Lying Triceps Extension: 3 hard sets	×	×	×
Weighted Sit-Up : 3 hard sets	×	×	×

NOTES:

WORKOUT 3: PULL			
EXERCISES	**SETS**		
Barbell Deadlift: Warm-up and 3 hard sets	×	×	×
Barbell Row: 3 hard sets	×	×	×
Seated Cable Row (Close-Grip): 3 hard sets	×	×	×
E-Z Bar Curl: 3 hard sets	×	×	×

NOTES:

_____

_____

_____

WORKOUT 4: LOWER BODY (LEGS AND GLUTES)			
EXERCISES	**SETS**		
Barbell Squat: Warm-up and 3 hard sets	×	×	×
Barbell Lunge (In-Place): 3 hard sets	×	×	×
Leg Curl (Lying or Seated)*: 3 hard sets	×	×	×
Glute Blaster: 3 hard sets	×	×	×

NOTES:

_____

_____

_____

| 4-DAY ROUTINE | PHASE 5 | WEEK 40 |

WORKOUT 1: LOWER BODY (LEGS AND GLUTES)

EXERCISES	SETS		
Barbell Squat: Warm-up and 3 hard sets	×	×	×
Barbell Single-Leg Split Squat : 3 hard sets	×	×	×
Romanian Deadlift: 3 hard sets	×	×	×
Hip Thrust: 3 hard sets	×	×	×

NOTES:

WORKOUT 2: UPPER BODY AND CORE

EXERCISES	SETS		
Barbell Bench Press: Warm-up and 3 hard sets	×	×	×
Dip: 3 hard sets	×	×	×
Barbell Rear Delt Row: 3 hard sets	×	×	×
Lying Triceps Extension: 3 hard sets	×	×	×
Weighted Sit-Up : 3 hard sets	×	×	×

NOTES:

WORKOUT 3: PULL			
EXERCISES	**SETS**		
Barbell Deadlift: Warm-up and 3 hard sets	×	×	×
Barbell Row: 3 hard sets	×	×	×
Seated Cable Row (Close-Grip): 3 hard sets	×	×	×
E-Z Bar Curl: 3 hard sets	×	×	×

NOTES:

WORKOUT 4: LOWER BODY (LEGS AND GLUTES)			
EXERCISES	**SETS**		
Barbell Squat: Warm-up and 3 hard sets	×	×	×
Barbell Lunge (In-Place): 3 hard sets	×	×	×
Leg Curl (Lying or Seated)*: 3 hard sets	×	×	×
Glute Blaster: 3 hard sets	×	×	×

NOTES:

4-DAY ROUTINE | PHASE 5 | WEEK 41

WORKOUT 1: LOWER BODY (LEGS AND GLUTES)

EXERCISES	SETS		
Barbell Squat: Warm-up and 3 hard sets	×	×	×
Barbell Single-Leg Split Squat : 3 hard sets	×	×	×
Romanian Deadlift: 3 hard sets	×	×	×
Hip Thrust: 3 hard sets	×	×	×

NOTES:

WORKOUT 2: UPPER BODY AND CORE

EXERCISES	SETS		
Barbell Bench Press: Warm-up and 3 hard sets	×	×	×
Dip: 3 hard sets	×	×	×
Barbell Rear Delt Row: 3 hard sets	×	×	×
Lying Triceps Extension: 3 hard sets	×	×	×
Weighted Sit-Up : 3 hard sets	×	×	×

NOTES:

WORKOUT 3: PULL			
EXERCISES	**SETS**		
Barbell Deadlift: Warm-up and 3 hard sets	×	×	×
Barbell Row: 3 hard sets	×	×	×
Seated Cable Row (Close-Grip): 3 hard sets	×	×	×
E-Z Bar Curl: 3 hard sets	×	×	×

NOTES:

_____

_____

_____

WORKOUT 4: LOWER BODY (LEGS AND GLUTES)			
EXERCISES	**SETS**		
Barbell Squat: Warm-up and 3 hard sets	×	×	×
Barbell Lunge (In-Place): 3 hard sets	×	×	×
Leg Curl (Lying or Seated)*: 3 hard sets	×	×	×
Glute Blaster: 3 hard sets	×	×	×

NOTES:

_____

_____

_____

| 4-DAY ROUTINE | PHASE 5 | WEEK 42 |

WORKOUT 1: LOWER BODY (LEGS AND GLUTES)

EXERCISES	SETS		
Barbell Squat: Warm-up and 3 hard sets	×	×	×
Barbell Single-Leg Split Squat : 3 hard sets	×	×	×
Romanian Deadlift: 3 hard sets	×	×	×
Hip Thrust: 3 hard sets	×	×	×

NOTES:

WORKOUT 2: UPPER BODY AND CORE

EXERCISES	SETS		
Barbell Bench Press: Warm-up and 3 hard sets	×	×	×
Dip: 3 hard sets	×	×	×
Barbell Rear Delt Row: 3 hard sets	×	×	×
Lying Triceps Extension: 3 hard sets	×	×	×
Weighted Sit-Up : 3 hard sets	×	×	×

NOTES:

WORKOUT 3: PULL			
EXERCISES	**SETS**		
Barbell Deadlift: Warm-up and 3 hard sets	×	×	×
Barbell Row: 3 hard sets	×	×	×
Seated Cable Row (Close-Grip): 3 hard sets	×	×	×
E-Z Bar Curl: 3 hard sets	×	×	×

NOTES:

_____

_____

WORKOUT 4: LOWER BODY (LEGS AND GLUTES)			
EXERCISES	**SETS**		
Barbell Squat: Warm-up and 3 hard sets	×	×	×
Barbell Lunge (In-Place): 3 hard sets	×	×	×
Leg Curl (Lying or Seated)*: 3 hard sets	×	×	×
Glute Blaster: 3 hard sets	×	×	×

NOTES:

_____

_____

4-DAY ROUTINE	PHASE 5	WEEK 43

WORKOUT 1: LOWER BODY (LEGS AND GLUTES)

EXERCISES	SETS		
Barbell Squat: Warm-up and 3 hard sets	×	×	×
Barbell Single-Leg Split Squat : 3 hard sets	×	×	×
Romanian Deadlift: 3 hard sets	×	×	×
Hip Thrust: 3 hard sets	×	×	×

NOTES:

_____

_____

WORKOUT 2: UPPER BODY AND CORE

EXERCISES	SETS		
Barbell Bench Press: Warm-up and 3 hard sets	×	×	×
Dip: 3 hard sets	×	×	×
Barbell Rear Delt Row: 3 hard sets	×	×	×
Lying Triceps Extension: 3 hard sets	×	×	×
Weighted Sit-Up : 3 hard sets	×	×	×

NOTES:

_____

_____

WORKOUT 3: PULL			
EXERCISES	**SETS**		
Barbell Deadlift: Warm-up and 3 hard sets	×	×	×
Barbell Row: 3 hard sets	×	×	×
Seated Cable Row (Close-Grip): 3 hard sets	×	×	×
E-Z Bar Curl: 3 hard sets	×	×	×

NOTES:

_____

_____

_____

WORKOUT 4: LOWER BODY (LEGS AND GLUTES)			
EXERCISES	**SETS**		
Barbell Squat: Warm-up and 3 hard sets	×	×	×
Barbell Lunge (In-Place): 3 hard sets	×	×	×
Leg Curl (Lying or Seated)*: 3 hard sets	×	×	×
Glute Blaster: 3 hard sets	×	×	×

NOTES:

_____

_____

_____

4-DAY ROUTINE	PHASE 5	WEEK 44

WORKOUT 1: LOWER BODY (LEGS AND GLUTES)

EXERCISES	SETS		
Barbell Squat: Warm-up and 3 hard sets	×	×	×
Barbell Single-Leg Split Squat : 3 hard sets	×	×	×
Romanian Deadlift: 3 hard sets	×	×	×
Hip Thrust: 3 hard sets	×	×	×

NOTES:

_____

_____

_____

WORKOUT 2: UPPER BODY AND CORE

EXERCISES	SETS		
Barbell Bench Press: Warm-up and 3 hard sets	×	×	×
Dip: 3 hard sets	×	×	×
Barbell Rear Delt Row: 3 hard sets	×	×	×
Lying Triceps Extension: 3 hard sets	×	×	×
Weighted Sit-Up : 3 hard sets	×	×	×

NOTES:

_____

_____

_____

WORKOUT 3: PULL			
EXERCISES	**SETS**		
Barbell Deadlift: Warm-up and 3 hard sets	×	×	×
Barbell Row: 3 hard sets	×	×	×
Seated Cable Row (Close-Grip): 3 hard sets	×	×	×
E-Z Bar Curl: 3 hard sets	×	×	×

NOTES:

WORKOUT 4: LOWER BODY (LEGS AND GLUTES)			
EXERCISES	**SETS**		
Barbell Squat: Warm-up and 3 hard sets	×	×	×
Barbell Lunge (In-Place): 3 hard sets	×	×	×
Leg Curl (Lying or Seated)*: 3 hard sets	×	×	×
Glute Blaster: 3 hard sets	×	×	×

NOTES:

4-DAY ROUTINE	DELOAD	WEEK 45

WORKOUT 1: DELOAD LEGS

EXERCISES	SETS		
Barbell Squat: Warm-up and 3 sets of 5 reps with last hard set weight	×	×	×
Romanian Deadlift: 3 sets of 5 reps with last hard set weight	×	×	×
Hip Thrust: 3 sets of 5 reps with last hard set weight	×	×	×

NOTES:

WORKOUT 2: DELOAD PUSH

EXERCISES	SETS		
Barbell Bench Press: Warm-up and 3 sets of 5 reps with last hard set weight	×	×	×
Seated Dumbbell Press: 3 sets of 5 reps with last hard set weight	×	×	×
Dumbbell Bench Press: 3 sets of 5 reps with last hard set weight	×	×	×

NOTES:

WORKOUT 3: DELOAD PULL

EXERCISES	SETS		
Barbell Deadlift: Warm-up and 3 sets of 5 reps with last hard set weight	×	×	×
Barbell Row: 3 sets of 5 reps with last hard set weight	×	×	×
Lat Pulldown (Wide-Grip): 3 sets of 5 reps with last hard set weight	×	×	×

NOTES:

3-DAY ROUTINE	PHASE 5	WEEK 37

WORKOUT 1: LOWER BODY (LEGS AND GLUTES)			
EXERCISES	**SETS**		
Barbell Squat: Warm-up and 3 hard sets	×	×	×
Barbell Single-Leg Split Squat : 3 hard sets	×	×	×
Romanian Deadlift: 3 hard sets	×	×	×
Hip Thrust: 3 hard sets	×	×	×

NOTES:

WORKOUT 2: UPPER BODY AND CORE			
EXERCISES	**SETS**		
Barbell Bench Press: Warm-up and 3 hard sets	×	×	×
Dip: 3 hard sets	×	×	×
Dumbbell Side Lateral Raise: 3 hard sets	×	×	×
Lying Triceps Extension: 3 hard sets	×	×	×
Hanging Leg Raise: 3 hard sets			

NOTES:

LOWER BODY AND PULL (LEGS AND BACK)			
EXERCISES	**SETS**		
Barbell Squat: Warm-up and 3 hard sets	×	×	×
Barbell Deadlift: Warm-up and 3 hard sets	×	×	×
Barbell Row: 3 hard sets	×	×	×
Chin-Up: 3 hard sets	×	×	×
Dumbbell Hammer Curl: 3 hard sets	×	×	×

NOTES:

3-DAY ROUTINE	PHASE 5	WEEK 38

WORKOUT 1: LOWER BODY (LEGS AND GLUTES)

EXERCISES	SETS		
Barbell Squat: Warm-up and 3 hard sets	×	×	×
Barbell Single-Leg Split Squat : 3 hard sets	×	×	×
Romanian Deadlift: 3 hard sets	×	×	×
Hip Thrust: 3 hard sets	×	×	×

NOTES:

WORKOUT 2: UPPER BODY AND CORE

EXERCISES	SETS		
Barbell Bench Press: Warm-up and 3 hard sets	×	×	×
Dip: 3 hard sets	×	×	×
Dumbbell Side Lateral Raise: 3 hard sets	×	×	×
Lying Triceps Extension: 3 hard sets	×	×	×
Hanging Leg Raise: 3 hard sets			

NOTES:

LOWER BODY AND PULL (LEGS AND BACK)

EXERCISES	SETS		
Barbell Squat: Warm-up and 3 hard sets	×	×	×
Barbell Deadlift: Warm-up and 3 hard sets	×	×	×
Barbell Row: 3 hard sets	×	×	×
Chin-Up: 3 hard sets	×	×	×
Dumbbell Hammer Curl: 3 hard sets	×	×	×

NOTES:

3-DAY ROUTINE	PHASE 5	WEEK 39

WORKOUT 1: LOWER BODY (LEGS AND GLUTES)			
EXERCISES	**SETS**		
Barbell Squat: Warm-up and 3 hard sets	×	×	×
Barbell Single-Leg Split Squat : 3 hard sets	×	×	×
Romanian Deadlift: 3 hard sets	×	×	×
Hip Thrust: 3 hard sets	×	×	×

NOTES:

WORKOUT 2: UPPER BODY AND CORE			
EXERCISES	**SETS**		
Barbell Bench Press: Warm-up and 3 hard sets	×	×	×
Dip: 3 hard sets	×	×	×
Dumbbell Side Lateral Raise: 3 hard sets	×	×	×
Lying Triceps Extension: 3 hard sets	×	×	×
Hanging Leg Raise: 3 hard sets			

NOTES:

LOWER BODY AND PULL (LEGS AND BACK)			
EXERCISES	**SETS**		
Barbell Squat: Warm-up and 3 hard sets	×	×	×
Barbell Deadlift: Warm-up and 3 hard sets	×	×	×
Barbell Row: 3 hard sets	×	×	×
Chin-Up: 3 hard sets	×	×	×
Dumbbell Hammer Curl: 3 hard sets	×	×	×

NOTES:

3-DAY ROUTINE | PHASE 5 | WEEK 40

WORKOUT 1: LOWER BODY (LEGS AND GLUTES)

EXERCISES	SETS		
Barbell Squat: Warm-up and 3 hard sets	×	×	×
Barbell Single-Leg Split Squat : 3 hard sets	×	×	×
Romanian Deadlift: 3 hard sets	×	×	×
Hip Thrust: 3 hard sets	×	×	×

NOTES:

WORKOUT 2: UPPER BODY AND CORE

EXERCISES	SETS		
Barbell Bench Press: Warm-up and 3 hard sets	×	×	×
Dip: 3 hard sets	×	×	×
Dumbbell Side Lateral Raise: 3 hard sets	×	×	×
Lying Triceps Extension: 3 hard sets	×	×	×
Hanging Leg Raise: 3 hard sets			

NOTES:

LOWER BODY AND PULL (LEGS AND BACK)

EXERCISES	SETS		
Barbell Squat: Warm-up and 3 hard sets	×	×	×
Barbell Deadlift: Warm-up and 3 hard sets	×	×	×
Barbell Row: 3 hard sets	×	×	×
Chin-Up: 3 hard sets	×	×	×
Dumbbell Hammer Curl: 3 hard sets	×	×	×

NOTES:

3-DAY ROUTINE	PHASE 5	WEEK 41

WORKOUT 1: LOWER BODY (LEGS AND GLUTES)			
EXERCISES	SETS		
Barbell Squat: Warm-up and 3 hard sets	×	×	×
Barbell Single-Leg Split Squat : 3 hard sets	×	×	×
Romanian Deadlift: 3 hard sets	×	×	×
Hip Thrust: 3 hard sets	×	×	×

NOTES:

WORKOUT 2: UPPER BODY AND CORE			
EXERCISES	SETS		
Barbell Bench Press: Warm-up and 3 hard sets	×	×	×
Dip: 3 hard sets	×	×	×
Dumbbell Side Lateral Raise: 3 hard sets	×	×	×
Lying Triceps Extension: 3 hard sets	×	×	×
Hanging Leg Raise: 3 hard sets			

NOTES:

LOWER BODY AND PULL (LEGS AND BACK)			
EXERCISES	SETS		
Barbell Squat: Warm-up and 3 hard sets	×	×	×
Barbell Deadlift: Warm-up and 3 hard sets	×	×	×
Barbell Row: 3 hard sets	×	×	×
Chin-Up: 3 hard sets	×	×	×
Dumbbell Hammer Curl: 3 hard sets	×	×	×

NOTES:

3-DAY ROUTINE	PHASE 5	WEEK 42

WORKOUT 1: LOWER BODY (LEGS AND GLUTES)

EXERCISES	SETS		
Barbell Squat: Warm-up and 3 hard sets	×	×	×
Barbell Single-Leg Split Squat : 3 hard sets	×	×	×
Romanian Deadlift: 3 hard sets	×	×	×
Hip Thrust: 3 hard sets	×	×	×

NOTES:

WORKOUT 2: UPPER BODY AND CORE

EXERCISES	SETS		
Barbell Bench Press: Warm-up and 3 hard sets	×	×	×
Dip: 3 hard sets	×	×	×
Dumbbell Side Lateral Raise: 3 hard sets	×	×	×
Lying Triceps Extension: 3 hard sets	×	×	×
Hanging Leg Raise: 3 hard sets			

NOTES:

LOWER BODY AND PULL (LEGS AND BACK)

EXERCISES	SETS		
Barbell Squat: Warm-up and 3 hard sets	×	×	×
Barbell Deadlift: Warm-up and 3 hard sets	×	×	×
Barbell Row: 3 hard sets	×	×	×
Chin-Up: 3 hard sets	×	×	×
Dumbbell Hammer Curl: 3 hard sets	×	×	×

NOTES:

3-DAY ROUTINE	PHASE 5	WEEK 43

WORKOUT 1: LOWER BODY (LEGS AND GLUTES)

EXERCISES	SETS		
Barbell Squat: Warm-up and 3 hard sets	×	×	×
Barbell Single-Leg Split Squat : 3 hard sets	×	×	×
Romanian Deadlift: 3 hard sets	×	×	×
Hip Thrust: 3 hard sets	×	×	×

NOTES:

WORKOUT 2: UPPER BODY AND CORE

EXERCISES	SETS		
Barbell Bench Press: Warm-up and 3 hard sets	×	×	×
Dip: 3 hard sets	×	×	×
Dumbbell Side Lateral Raise: 3 hard sets	×	×	×
Lying Triceps Extension: 3 hard sets	×	×	×
Hanging Leg Raise: 3 hard sets			

NOTES:

LOWER BODY AND PULL (LEGS AND BACK)

EXERCISES	SETS		
Barbell Squat: Warm-up and 3 hard sets	×	×	×
Barbell Deadlift: Warm-up and 3 hard sets	×	×	×
Barbell Row: 3 hard sets	×	×	×
Chin-Up: 3 hard sets	×	×	×
Dumbbell Hammer Curl: 3 hard sets	×	×	×

NOTES:

3-DAY ROUTINE | PHASE 5 | WEEK 44

WORKOUT 1: LOWER BODY (LEGS AND GLUTES)

EXERCISES	SETS		
Barbell Squat: Warm-up and 3 hard sets	×	×	×
Barbell Single-Leg Split Squat : 3 hard sets	×	×	×
Romanian Deadlift: 3 hard sets	×	×	×
Hip Thrust: 3 hard sets	×	×	×

NOTES:

WORKOUT 2: UPPER BODY AND CORE

EXERCISES	SETS		
Barbell Bench Press: Warm-up and 3 hard sets	×	×	×
Dip: 3 hard sets	×	×	×
Dumbbell Side Lateral Raise: 3 hard sets	×	×	×
Lying Triceps Extension: 3 hard sets	×	×	×
Hanging Leg Raise: 3 hard sets			

NOTES:

LOWER BODY AND PULL (LEGS AND BACK)

EXERCISES	SETS		
Barbell Squat: Warm-up and 3 hard sets	×	×	×
Barbell Deadlift: Warm-up and 3 hard sets	×	×	×
Barbell Row: 3 hard sets	×	×	×
Chin-Up: 3 hard sets	×	×	×
Dumbbell Hammer Curl: 3 hard sets	×	×	×

NOTES:

3-DAY ROUTINE	DELOAD	WEEK 45

WORKOUT 1: DELOAD LEGS			
EXERCISES	**SETS**		
Barbell Squat: Warm-up and 3 sets of 5 reps with last hard set weight	×	×	×
Romanian Deadlift: 3 sets of 5 reps with last hard set weight	×	×	×
Hip Thrust: 3 sets of 5 reps with last hard set weight	×	×	×

NOTES:

WORKOUT 2: DELOAD PUSH			
EXERCISES	**SETS**		
Barbell Bench Press: Warm-up and 3 sets of 5 reps with last hard set weight	×	×	×
Seated Dumbbell Press: 3 sets of 5 reps with last hard set weight	×	×	×
Dumbbell Bench Press: 3 sets of 5 reps with last hard set weight	×	×	×

NOTES:

WORKOUT 3: DELOAD PULL			
EXERCISES	**SETS**		
Barbell Deadlift: Warm-up and 3 sets of 5 reps with last hard set weight	×	×	×
Barbell Row: 3 sets of 5 reps with last hard set weight	×	×	×
Lat Pulldown (Wide-Grip): 3 sets of 5 reps with last hard set weight	×	×	×

NOTES:

Do you see that in the distance?

The huge, shiny object full of angels and chocolate coins?

What is that?

Oh that's right, it's the trophy you're going to get when you finish the next and final phase of this program!

At that point, you'll be able to proudly say that you've invested an entire year into your health, fitness, and well-being. I don't know about you, but I can't wait until you cross that finish line!

And that's not all we have to be excited about, either.

By now your strength should be over the roof in comparison to where you started, and you have a real idea of just how good you can look in the mirror with a bit of know-how and elbow grease.

Feels good, doesn't it? The best part is that it will just keep getting better and better—for a long time to come.

You're just a couple months away from finishing the Year One Challenge for Women, so let's take new measurements and pictures, and come flying out of the gates into your final lap.

First, take the following body measurements first thing in the morning, nude, after using the bathroom and before eating or drinking anything:

1. Weight

2. Waist circumference

3. OPTIONAL: Hip circumference

4. OPTIONAL: Upper-leg circumference

5. OPTIONAL: Flexed arms

Then, take flexed and unflexed pictures from the front, back, and sides, and store them in an album or folder that you can easily locate later.

Remember to show as much skin as you feel comfortable with. The more the better because it will give you the best idea of how your body is responding to the program.

DON'T SACRIFICE WHO YOU COULD BE FOR WHO YOU ARE.

—DR. JORDAN PETERSON

THINNER LEANER STRONGER PHASE 6

You've reached the final phase of the *Year One Challenge for Women.*

That means that you've accomplished what many women only dream of. You've worked your butt off for 10 months now, and you have a whole new body to show for it.

You've gained a bunch of lean muscle, lost a bunch of unwanted fat, and are probably far stronger now than you've ever been before. I'll bet that family and friends who haven't seen you in a while can't believe their eyes!

And you know what? You're just getting started. You have a lot more fun ahead of you. In fact, you literally have the rest of your life to sculpt and mold your body into whatever you want it to be.

So, on the following pages, you'll find your next nine weeks of Thinner Leaner Stronger training. And once you've completed them, you'll have completed your very first year. Bask in that for a minute.

As before, choose the split that best suits your goals and circumstances, and stick with it until you've completed this sixth phase.

Answer the following questions, and if you have a lot to say, jot it down so you can easily refer back to it.

→ What are three things in your diet and/or training that went particularly well in the last phase? Why?

→ What's one thing you could have done better? Why?

→ What's one thing you can do to make your next phase even better than the last?

Okay, so now are you ready to get into the gym to pick up some heavy stuff and put it back down!? Excited!?

Let's go!

5-DAY ROUTINE	PHASE 6	WEEK 46

WORKOUT 1: LOWER BODY (LEGS AND GLUTES)			
EXERCISES	**SETS**		
Barbell Squat: Warm-up and 3 hard sets	×	×	×
Barbell Lunge (Walking): 3 hard sets	×	×	×
Leg Curl (Lying or Seated)*: 3 hard sets	×	×	×
Dumbbell Step-Up: 3 hard sets	×	×	×

NOTES:

WORKOUT 2: PUSH AND CORE			
EXERCISES	**SETS**		
Barbell Bench Press: Warm-up and 3 hard sets	×	×	×
Dumbbell Bench Press: 3 hard sets	×	×	×
Dip: 3 hard sets	×	×	×
Dumbbell Rear Lateral Raise (Bent-Over): 3 hard sets	×	×	×
Weighted Sit-Up: 3 hard sets	×	×	×

NOTES:

WORKOUT 3: PULL			
EXERCISES	**SETS**		
Barbell Deadlift: Warm-up and 3 hard sets	×	×	×
Pull-Up: 3 hard sets	×	×	×
Lat Pulldown (Wide-Grip): 3 hard sets	×	×	×
Alternating Dumbbell Curl: 3 hard sets	×	×	×

NOTES:

WORKOUT 4: UPPER BODY AND CORE			
EXERCISES	**SETS**		
Arnold Dumbbell Press: Warm-up and 3 hard sets	×	×	×
Close-Grip Bench Press: 3 hard sets	×	×	×
Dumbbell Side Lateral Raise: 3 hard sets	×	×	×
Triceps Pushdown: 3 hard sets	×	×	×
Hanging Leg Raise: 3 hard sets			

NOTES:

WORKOUT 5: LOWER BODY (LEGS AND GLUTES)			
EXERCISES	**SETS**		
Barbell Front Squat: Warm-up and 3 hard sets	×	×	×
Dumbbell Lunge (Reverse): 3 hard sets	×	×	×
Romanian Deadlift: 3 hard sets	×	×	×
Hip Thrust: 3 hard sets	×	×	×

NOTES:

5-DAY ROUTINE	PHASE 6	WEEK 47

WORKOUT 1: LOWER BODY (LEGS AND GLUTES)			
EXERCISES	**SETS**		
Barbell Squat: Warm-up and 3 hard sets	×	×	×
Barbell Lunge (Walking): 3 hard sets	×	×	×
Leg Curl (Lying or Seated)*: 3 hard sets	×	×	×
Dumbbell Step-Up: 3 hard sets	×	×	×

NOTES:

WORKOUT 2: PUSH AND CORE			
EXERCISES	**SETS**		
Barbell Bench Press: Warm-up and 3 hard sets	×	×	×
Dumbbell Bench Press: 3 hard sets	×	×	×
Dip: 3 hard sets	×	×	×
Dumbbell Rear Lateral Raise (Bent-Over): 3 hard sets	×	×	×
Weighted Sit-Up: 3 hard sets	×	×	×

NOTES:

WORKOUT 3: PULL			
EXERCISES	**SETS**		
Barbell Deadlift: Warm-up and 3 hard sets	×	×	×
Pull-Up: 3 hard sets	×	×	×
Lat Pulldown (Wide-Grip): 3 hard sets	×	×	×
Alternating Dumbbell Curl: 3 hard sets	×	×	×

NOTES:

WORKOUT 4: UPPER BODY AND CORE			
EXERCISES	**SETS**		
Arnold Dumbbell Press: Warm-up and 3 hard sets	×	×	×
Close-Grip Bench Press: 3 hard sets	×	×	×
Dumbbell Side Lateral Raise: 3 hard sets	×	×	×
Triceps Pushdown: 3 hard sets	×	×	×
Hanging Leg Raise: 3 hard sets			

NOTES:

WORKOUT 5: LOWER BODY (LEGS AND GLUTES)			
EXERCISES	**SETS**		
Barbell Front Squat: Warm-up and 3 hard sets	×	×	×
Dumbbell Lunge (Reverse): 3 hard sets	×	×	×
Romanian Deadlift: 3 hard sets	×	×	×
Hip Thrust: 3 hard sets	×	×	×

NOTES:

5-DAY ROUTINE	PHASE 6	WEEK 48

WORKOUT 1: LOWER BODY (LEGS AND GLUTES)

EXERCISES	SETS		
Barbell Squat: Warm-up and 3 hard sets	×	×	×
Barbell Lunge (Walking): 3 hard sets	×	×	×
Leg Curl (Lying or Seated)*: 3 hard sets	×	×	×
Dumbbell Step-Up: 3 hard sets	×	×	×

NOTES:

WORKOUT 2: PUSH AND CORE

EXERCISES	SETS		
Barbell Bench Press: Warm-up and 3 hard sets	×	×	×
Dumbbell Bench Press: 3 hard sets	×	×	×
Dip: 3 hard sets	×	×	×
Dumbbell Rear Lateral Raise (Bent-Over): 3 hard sets	×	×	×
Weighted Sit-Up: 3 hard sets	×	×	×

NOTES:

WORKOUT 3: PULL

EXERCISES	SETS		
Barbell Deadlift: Warm-up and 3 hard sets	×	×	×
Pull-Up: 3 hard sets	×	×	×
Lat Pulldown (Wide-Grip): 3 hard sets	×	×	×
Alternating Dumbbell Curl: 3 hard sets	×	×	×

NOTES:

WORKOUT 4: UPPER BODY AND CORE			
EXERCISES	**SETS**		
Arnold Dumbbell Press: Warm-up and 3 hard sets	×	×	×
Close-Grip Bench Press: 3 hard sets	×	×	×
Dumbbell Side Lateral Raise: 3 hard sets	×	×	×
Triceps Pushdown: 3 hard sets	×	×	×
Hanging Leg Raise: 3 hard sets			

NOTES:

_____

_____

_____

WORKOUT 5: LOWER BODY (LEGS AND GLUTES)			
EXERCISES	**SETS**		
Barbell Front Squat: Warm-up and 3 hard sets	×	×	×
Dumbbell Lunge (Reverse): 3 hard sets	×	×	×
Romanian Deadlift: 3 hard sets	×	×	×
Hip Thrust: 3 hard sets	×	×	×

NOTES:

_____

_____

5-DAY ROUTINE	PHASE 6	WEEK 49

WORKOUT 1: LOWER BODY (LEGS AND GLUTES)			
EXERCISES	**SETS**		
Barbell Squat: Warm-up and 3 hard sets	×	×	×
Barbell Lunge (Walking): 3 hard sets	×	×	×
Leg Curl (Lying or Seated)*: 3 hard sets	×	×	×
Dumbbell Step-Up: 3 hard sets	×	×	×

NOTES:

WORKOUT 2: PUSH AND CORE			
EXERCISES	**SETS**		
Barbell Bench Press: Warm-up and 3 hard sets	×	×	×
Dumbbell Bench Press: 3 hard sets	×	×	×
Dip: 3 hard sets	×	×	×
Dumbbell Rear Lateral Raise (Bent-Over): 3 hard sets	×	×	×
Weighted Sit-Up: 3 hard sets	×	×	×

NOTES:

WORKOUT 3: PULL			
EXERCISES	**SETS**		
Barbell Deadlift: Warm-up and 3 hard sets	×	×	×
Pull-Up: 3 hard sets	×	×	×
Lat Pulldown (Wide-Grip): 3 hard sets	×	×	×
Alternating Dumbbell Curl: 3 hard sets	×	×	×

NOTES:

WORKOUT 4: UPPER BODY AND CORE			
EXERCISES	**SETS**		
Arnold Dumbbell Press: Warm-up and 3 hard sets	×	×	×
Close-Grip Bench Press: 3 hard sets	×	×	×
Dumbbell Side Lateral Raise: 3 hard sets	×	×	×
Triceps Pushdown: 3 hard sets	×	×	×
Hanging Leg Raise: 3 hard sets			

NOTES:

_____

_____

_____

WORKOUT 5: LOWER BODY (LEGS AND GLUTES)			
EXERCISES	**SETS**		
Barbell Front Squat: Warm-up and 3 hard sets	×	×	×
Dumbbell Lunge (Reverse): 3 hard sets	×	×	×
Romanian Deadlift: 3 hard sets	×	×	×
Hip Thrust: 3 hard sets	×	×	×

NOTES:

_____

_____

_____

| 5-DAY ROUTINE | PHASE 6 | WEEK 50 |

WORKOUT 1: LOWER BODY (LEGS AND GLUTES)			
EXERCISES	SETS		
Barbell Squat: Warm-up and 3 hard sets	×	×	×
Barbell Lunge (Walking): 3 hard sets	×	×	×
Leg Curl (Lying or Seated)*: 3 hard sets	×	×	×
Dumbbell Step-Up: 3 hard sets	×	×	×

NOTES:

WORKOUT 2: PUSH AND CORE			
EXERCISES	SETS		
Barbell Bench Press: Warm-up and 3 hard sets	×	×	×
Dumbbell Bench Press: 3 hard sets	×	×	×
Dip: 3 hard sets	×	×	×
Dumbbell Rear Lateral Raise (Bent-Over): 3 hard sets	×	×	×
Weighted Sit-Up: 3 hard sets	×	×	×

NOTES:

WORKOUT 3: PULL			
EXERCISES	SETS		
Barbell Deadlift: Warm-up and 3 hard sets	×	×	×
Pull-Up: 3 hard sets	×	×	×
Lat Pulldown (Wide-Grip): 3 hard sets	×	×	×
Alternating Dumbbell Curl: 3 hard sets	×	×	×

NOTES:

WORKOUT 4: UPPER BODY AND CORE			
EXERCISES	**SETS**		
Arnold Dumbbell Press: Warm-up and 3 hard sets	×	×	×
Close-Grip Bench Press: 3 hard sets	×	×	×
Dumbbell Side Lateral Raise: 3 hard sets	×	×	×
Triceps Pushdown: 3 hard sets	×	×	×
Hanging Leg Raise: 3 hard sets			

NOTES:

_____

_____

_____

WORKOUT 5: LOWER BODY (LEGS AND GLUTES)			
EXERCISES	**SETS**		
Barbell Front Squat: Warm-up and 3 hard sets	×	×	×
Dumbbell Lunge (Reverse): 3 hard sets	×	×	×
Romanian Deadlift: 3 hard sets	×	×	×
Hip Thrust: 3 hard sets	×	×	×

NOTES:

_____

_____

_____

5-DAY ROUTINE	PHASE 6	WEEK 51

WORKOUT 1: LOWER BODY (LEGS AND GLUTES)			
EXERCISES	SETS		
Barbell Squat: Warm-up and 3 hard sets	×	×	×
Barbell Lunge (Walking): 3 hard sets	×	×	×
Leg Curl (Lying or Seated)*: 3 hard sets	×	×	×
Dumbbell Step-Up: 3 hard sets	×	×	×

NOTES:

WORKOUT 2: PUSH AND CORE			
EXERCISES	SETS		
Barbell Bench Press: Warm-up and 3 hard sets	×	×	×
Dumbbell Bench Press: 3 hard sets	×	×	×
Dip: 3 hard sets	×	×	×
Dumbbell Rear Lateral Raise (Bent-Over): 3 hard sets	×	×	×
Weighted Sit-Up: 3 hard sets	×	×	×

NOTES:

WORKOUT 3: PULL			
EXERCISES	SETS		
Barbell Deadlift: Warm-up and 3 hard sets	×	×	×
Pull-Up: 3 hard sets	×	×	×
Lat Pulldown (Wide-Grip): 3 hard sets	×	×	×
Alternating Dumbbell Curl: 3 hard sets	×	×	×

NOTES:

WORKOUT 4: UPPER BODY AND CORE			
EXERCISES	**SETS**		
Arnold Dumbbell Press: Warm-up and 3 hard sets	×	×	×
Close-Grip Bench Press: 3 hard sets	×	×	×
Dumbbell Side Lateral Raise: 3 hard sets	×	×	×
Triceps Pushdown: 3 hard sets	×	×	×
Hanging Leg Raise: 3 hard sets			

NOTES:

_____

_____

_____

WORKOUT 5: LOWER BODY (LEGS AND GLUTES)			
EXERCISES	**SETS**		
Barbell Front Squat: Warm-up and 3 hard sets	×	×	×
Dumbbell Lunge (Reverse): 3 hard sets	×	×	×
Romanian Deadlift: 3 hard sets	×	×	×
Hip Thrust: 3 hard sets	×	×	×

NOTES:

_____

_____

_____

5-DAY ROUTINE	PHASE 6	WEEK 52

WORKOUT 1: LOWER BODY (LEGS AND GLUTES)			
EXERCISES	**SETS**		
Barbell Squat: Warm-up and 3 hard sets	×	×	×
Barbell Lunge (Walking): 3 hard sets	×	×	×
Leg Curl (Lying or Seated)*: 3 hard sets	×	×	×
Dumbbell Step-Up: 3 hard sets	×	×	×

NOTES:

WORKOUT 2: PUSH AND CORE			
EXERCISES	**SETS**		
Barbell Bench Press: Warm-up and 3 hard sets	×	×	×
Dumbbell Bench Press: 3 hard sets	×	×	×
Dip: 3 hard sets	×	×	×
Dumbbell Rear Lateral Raise (Bent-Over): 3 hard sets	×	×	×
Weighted Sit-Up: 3 hard sets	×	×	×

NOTES:

WORKOUT 3: PULL			
EXERCISES	**SETS**		
Barbell Deadlift: Warm-up and 3 hard sets	×	×	×
Pull-Up: 3 hard sets	×	×	×
Lat Pulldown (Wide-Grip): 3 hard sets	×	×	×
Alternating Dumbbell Curl: 3 hard sets	×	×	×

NOTES:

WORKOUT 4: UPPER BODY AND CORE			
EXERCISES	**SETS**		
Arnold Dumbbell Press: Warm-up and 3 hard sets	×	×	×
Close-Grip Bench Press: 3 hard sets	×	×	×
Dumbbell Side Lateral Raise: 3 hard sets	×	×	×
Triceps Pushdown: 3 hard sets	×	×	×
Hanging Leg Raise: 3 hard sets			

NOTES:

_____

_____

_____

WORKOUT 5: LOWER BODY (LEGS AND GLUTES)			
EXERCISES	**SETS**		
Barbell Front Squat: Warm-up and 3 hard sets	×	×	×
Dumbbell Lunge (Reverse): 3 hard sets	×	×	×
Romanian Deadlift: 3 hard sets	×	×	×
Hip Thrust: 3 hard sets	×	×	×

NOTES:

_____

_____

_____

5-DAY ROUTINE	PHASE 6	WEEK 53

WORKOUT 1: LOWER BODY (LEGS AND GLUTES)			
EXERCISES	SETS		
Barbell Squat: Warm-up and 3 hard sets	×	×	×
Barbell Lunge (Walking): 3 hard sets	×	×	×
Leg Curl (Lying or Seated)*: 3 hard sets	×	×	×
Dumbbell Step-Up: 3 hard sets	×	×	×

NOTES:

WORKOUT 2: PUSH AND CORE			
EXERCISES	SETS		
Barbell Bench Press: Warm-up and 3 hard sets	×	×	×
Dumbbell Bench Press: 3 hard sets	×	×	×
Dip: 3 hard sets	×	×	×
Dumbbell Rear Lateral Raise (Bent-Over): 3 hard sets	×	×	×
Weighted Sit-Up: 3 hard sets	×	×	×

NOTES:

WORKOUT 3: PULL			
EXERCISES	SETS		
Barbell Deadlift: Warm-up and 3 hard sets	×	×	×
Pull-Up: 3 hard sets	×	×	×
Lat Pulldown (Wide-Grip): 3 hard sets	×	×	×
Alternating Dumbbell Curl: 3 hard sets	×	×	×

NOTES:

WORKOUT 4: UPPER BODY AND CORE			
EXERCISES	SETS		
Arnold Dumbbell Press: Warm-up and 3 hard sets	×	×	×
Close-Grip Bench Press: 3 hard sets	×	×	×
Dumbbell Side Lateral Raise: 3 hard sets	×	×	×
Triceps Pushdown: 3 hard sets	×	×	×
Hanging Leg Raise: 3 hard sets			

NOTES:

WORKOUT 5: LOWER BODY (LEGS AND GLUTES)			
EXERCISES	SETS		
Barbell Front Squat: Warm-up and 3 hard sets	×	×	×
Dumbbell Lunge (Reverse): 3 hard sets	×	×	×
Romanian Deadlift: 3 hard sets	×	×	×
Hip Thrust: 3 hard sets	×	×	×

NOTES:

5-DAY ROUTINE	DELOAD	WEEK 54

WORKOUT 1: DELOAD LEGS

EXERCISES		SETS	
Barbell Squat: Warm-up and 3 sets of 5 reps with last hard set weight	×	×	×
Romanian Deadlift: 3 sets of 5 reps with last hard set weight	×	×	×
Hip Thrust: 3 sets of 5 reps with last hard set weight	×	×	×

NOTES:

WORKOUT 2: DELOAD PUSH

EXERCISES		SETS	
Barbell Bench Press: Warm-up and 3 sets of 5 reps with last hard set weight	×	×	×
Seated Dumbbell Press: 3 sets of 5 reps with last hard set weight	×	×	×
Dumbbell Side Lateral Raise: 3 sets of 5 reps with last hard set weight	×	×	×

NOTES:

WORKOUT 3: DELOAD PULL

EXERCISES		SETS	
Barbell Deadlift: Warm-up and 3 sets of 5 reps with last hard set weight	×	×	×
Barbell Row: 3 sets of 5 reps with last hard set weight	×	×	×
Lat Pulldown (Wide-Grip): 3 sets of 5 reps with last hard set weight	×	×	×

NOTES:

4-DAY ROUTINE	PHASE 6	WEEK 46

WORKOUT 1: LOWER BODY (LEGS AND GLUTES)

EXERCISES	SETS		
Barbell Squat: Warm-up and 3 hard sets	×	×	×
Barbell Lunge (Walking): 3 hard sets	×	×	×
Leg Curl (Lying or Seated)*: 3 hard sets	×	×	×
Dumbbell Step-Up: 3 hard sets	×	×	×

NOTES:

WORKOUT 2: UPPER BODY AND CORE

EXERCISES	SETS		
Barbell Bench Press: Warm-up and 3 hard sets	×	×	×
Dip: 3 hard sets	×	×	×
Dumbbell Rear Lateral Raise (Bent-Over): 3 hard sets	×	×	×
Triceps Pushdown: 3 hard sets	×	×	×
Hanging Leg Raise: 3 hard sets			

NOTES:

WORKOUT 3: PULL			
EXERCISES	**SETS**		
Barbell Deadlift: Warm-up and 3 hard sets	×	×	×
Pull-Up: 3 hard sets	×	×	×
Lat Pulldown (Wide-Grip): 3 hard sets	×	×	×
Alternating Dumbbell Curl: 3 hard sets	×	×	×

NOTES:

WORKOUT 4: LOWER BODY (LEGS AND GLUTES)			
EXERCISES	**SETS**		
Barbell Squat: Warm-up and 3 hard sets	×	×	×
Dumbbell Lunge (Reverse): 3 hard sets	×	×	×
Romanian Deadlift: 3 hard sets	×	×	×
Hip Thrust: 3 hard sets	×	×	×

NOTES:

| 4-DAY ROUTINE | PHASE 6 | WEEK 47 |

WORKOUT 1: LOWER BODY (LEGS AND GLUTES)

EXERCISES	SETS		
Barbell Squat: Warm-up and 3 hard sets	×	×	×
Barbell Lunge (Walking): 3 hard sets	×	×	×
Leg Curl (Lying or Seated)*: 3 hard sets	×	×	×
Dumbbell Step-Up: 3 hard sets	×	×	×

NOTES:

WORKOUT 2: UPPER BODY AND CORE

EXERCISES	SETS		
Barbell Bench Press: Warm-up and 3 hard sets	×	×	×
Dip: 3 hard sets	×	×	×
Dumbbell Rear Lateral Raise (Bent-Over): 3 hard sets	×	×	×
Triceps Pushdown: 3 hard sets	×	×	×
Hanging Leg Raise: 3 hard sets			

NOTES:

WORKOUT 3: PULL			
EXERCISES	**SETS**		
Barbell Deadlift: Warm-up and 3 hard sets	✕	✕	✕
Pull-Up: 3 hard sets	✕	✕	✕
Lat Pulldown (Wide-Grip): 3 hard sets	✕	✕	✕
Alternating Dumbbell Curl: 3 hard sets	✕	✕	✕

NOTES:

_____

_____

_____

WORKOUT 4: LOWER BODY (LEGS AND GLUTES)			
EXERCISES	**SETS**		
Barbell Squat: Warm-up and 3 hard sets	✕	✕	✕
Dumbbell Lunge (Reverse): 3 hard sets	✕	✕	✕
Romanian Deadlift: 3 hard sets	✕	✕	✕
Hip Thrust: 3 hard sets	✕	✕	✕

NOTES:

_____

_____

_____

| 4-DAY ROUTINE | PHASE 6 | WEEK 48 |

WORKOUT 1: LOWER BODY (LEGS AND GLUTES)

EXERCISES	SETS		
Barbell Squat: Warm-up and 3 hard sets	×	×	×
Barbell Lunge (Walking): 3 hard sets	×	×	×
Leg Curl (Lying or Seated)*: 3 hard sets	×	×	×
Dumbbell Step-Up: 3 hard sets	×	×	×

NOTES:

WORKOUT 2: UPPER BODY AND CORE

EXERCISES	SETS		
Barbell Bench Press: Warm-up and 3 hard sets	×	×	×
Dip: 3 hard sets	×	×	×
Dumbbell Rear Lateral Raise (Bent-Over): 3 hard sets	×	×	×
Triceps Pushdown: 3 hard sets	×	×	×
Hanging Leg Raise: 3 hard sets			

NOTES:

WORKOUT 3: PULL			
EXERCISES	**SETS**		
Barbell Deadlift: Warm-up and 3 hard sets	×	×	×
Pull-Up: 3 hard sets	×	×	×
Lat Pulldown (Wide-Grip): 3 hard sets	×	×	×
Alternating Dumbbell Curl: 3 hard sets	×	×	×

NOTES:

WORKOUT 4: LOWER BODY (LEGS AND GLUTES)			
EXERCISES	**SETS**		
Barbell Squat: Warm-up and 3 hard sets	×	×	×
Dumbbell Lunge (Reverse): 3 hard sets	×	×	×
Romanian Deadlift: 3 hard sets	×	×	×
Hip Thrust: 3 hard sets	×	×	×

NOTES:

4-DAY ROUTINE	PHASE 6	WEEK 49

WORKOUT 1: LOWER BODY (LEGS AND GLUTES)

EXERCISES	SETS		
Barbell Squat: Warm-up and 3 hard sets	×	×	×
Barbell Lunge (Walking): 3 hard sets	×	×	×
Leg Curl (Lying or Seated)*: 3 hard sets	×	×	×
Dumbbell Step-Up: 3 hard sets	×	×	×

NOTES:

WORKOUT 2: UPPER BODY AND CORE

EXERCISES	SETS		
Barbell Bench Press: Warm-up and 3 hard sets	×	×	×
Dip: 3 hard sets	×	×	×
Dumbbell Rear Lateral Raise (Bent-Over): 3 hard sets	×	×	×
Triceps Pushdown: 3 hard sets	×	×	×
Hanging Leg Raise: 3 hard sets			

NOTES:

WORKOUT 3: PULL			
EXERCISES	**SETS**		
Barbell Deadlift: Warm-up and 3 hard sets	×	×	×
Pull-Up: 3 hard sets	×	×	×
Lat Pulldown (Wide-Grip): 3 hard sets	×	×	×
Alternating Dumbbell Curl: 3 hard sets	×	×	×

NOTES:

_____

_____

_____

WORKOUT 4: LOWER BODY (LEGS AND GLUTES)			
EXERCISES	**SETS**		
Barbell Squat: Warm-up and 3 hard sets	×	×	×
Dumbbell Lunge (Reverse): 3 hard sets	×	×	×
Romanian Deadlift: 3 hard sets	×	×	×
Hip Thrust: 3 hard sets	×	×	×

NOTES:

_____

_____

_____

| 4-DAY ROUTINE | PHASE 6 | WEEK 50 |

WORKOUT 1: LOWER BODY (LEGS AND GLUTES)

EXERCISES	SETS		
Barbell Squat: Warm-up and 3 hard sets	×	×	×
Barbell Lunge (Walking): 3 hard sets	×	×	×
Leg Curl (Lying or Seated)*: 3 hard sets	×	×	×
Dumbbell Step-Up: 3 hard sets	×	×	×

NOTES:

WORKOUT 2: UPPER BODY AND CORE

EXERCISES	SETS		
Barbell Bench Press: Warm-up and 3 hard sets	×	×	×
Dip: 3 hard sets	×	×	×
Dumbbell Rear Lateral Raise (Bent-Over): 3 hard sets	×	×	×
Triceps Pushdown: 3 hard sets	×	×	×
Hanging Leg Raise: 3 hard sets			

NOTES:

WORKOUT 3: PULL			
EXERCISES	SETS		
Barbell Deadlift: Warm-up and 3 hard sets	×	×	×
Pull-Up: 3 hard sets	×	×	×
Lat Pulldown (Wide-Grip): 3 hard sets	×	×	×
Alternating Dumbbell Curl: 3 hard sets	×	×	×

NOTES:

\
\
\

WORKOUT 4: LOWER BODY (LEGS AND GLUTES)			
EXERCISES	SETS		
Barbell Squat: Warm-up and 3 hard sets	×	×	×
Dumbbell Lunge (Reverse): 3 hard sets	×	×	×
Romanian Deadlift: 3 hard sets	×	×	×
Hip Thrust: 3 hard sets	×	×	×

NOTES:

4-DAY ROUTINE	PHASE 6	WEEK 51

WORKOUT 1: LOWER BODY (LEGS AND GLUTES)			
EXERCISES	**SETS**		
Barbell Squat: Warm-up and 3 hard sets	×	×	×
Barbell Lunge (Walking): 3 hard sets	×	×	×
Leg Curl (Lying or Seated)*: 3 hard sets	×	×	×
Dumbbell Step-Up: 3 hard sets	×	×	×

NOTES:

_____

_____

WORKOUT 2: UPPER BODY AND CORE			
EXERCISES	**SETS**		
Barbell Bench Press: Warm-up and 3 hard sets	×	×	×
Dip: 3 hard sets	×	×	×
Dumbbell Rear Lateral Raise (Bent-Over): 3 hard sets	×	×	×
Triceps Pushdown: 3 hard sets	×	×	×
Hanging Leg Raise: 3 hard sets			

NOTES:

_____

_____

WORKOUT 3: PULL			
EXERCISES	**SETS**		
Barbell Deadlift: Warm-up and 3 hard sets	×	×	×
Pull-Up: 3 hard sets	×	×	×
Lat Pulldown (Wide-Grip): 3 hard sets	×	×	×
Alternating Dumbbell Curl: 3 hard sets	×	×	×

NOTES:

_____

_____

_____

WORKOUT 4: LOWER BODY (LEGS AND GLUTES)			
EXERCISES	**SETS**		
Barbell Squat: Warm-up and 3 hard sets	×	×	×
Dumbbell Lunge (Reverse): 3 hard sets	×	×	×
Romanian Deadlift: 3 hard sets	×	×	×
Hip Thrust: 3 hard sets	×	×	×

NOTES:

_____

_____

_____

| 4-DAY ROUTINE | PHASE 6 | WEEK 52 |

WORKOUT 1: LOWER BODY (LEGS AND GLUTES)

EXERCISES	SETS		
Barbell Squat: Warm-up and 3 hard sets	×	×	×
Barbell Lunge (Walking): 3 hard sets	×	×	×
Leg Curl (Lying or Seated)*: 3 hard sets	×	×	×
Dumbbell Step-Up: 3 hard sets	×	×	×

NOTES:

WORKOUT 2: UPPER BODY AND CORE

EXERCISES	SETS		
Barbell Bench Press: Warm-up and 3 hard sets	×	×	×
Dip: 3 hard sets	×	×	×
Dumbbell Rear Lateral Raise (Bent-Over): 3 hard sets	×	×	×
Triceps Pushdown: 3 hard sets	×	×	×
Hanging Leg Raise: 3 hard sets			

NOTES:

WORKOUT 3: PULL			
EXERCISES	SETS		
Barbell Deadlift: Warm-up and 3 hard sets	×	×	×
Pull-Up: 3 hard sets	×	×	×
Lat Pulldown (Wide-Grip): 3 hard sets	×	×	×
Alternating Dumbbell Curl: 3 hard sets	×	×	×

NOTES:

WORKOUT 4: LOWER BODY (LEGS AND GLUTES)			
EXERCISES	SETS		
Barbell Squat: Warm-up and 3 hard sets	×	×	×
Dumbbell Lunge (Reverse): 3 hard sets	×	×	×
Romanian Deadlift: 3 hard sets	×	×	×
Hip Thrust: 3 hard sets	×	×	×

NOTES:

4-DAY ROUTINE	PHASE 6	WEEK 53

WORKOUT 1: LOWER BODY (LEGS AND GLUTES)

EXERCISES	SETS		
Barbell Squat: Warm-up and 3 hard sets	×	×	×
Barbell Lunge (Walking): 3 hard sets	×	×	×
Leg Curl (Lying or Seated)*: 3 hard sets	×	×	×
Dumbbell Step-Up: 3 hard sets	×	×	×

NOTES:

WORKOUT 2: UPPER BODY AND CORE

EXERCISES	SETS		
Barbell Bench Press: Warm-up and 3 hard sets	×	×	×
Dip: 3 hard sets	×	×	×
Dumbbell Rear Lateral Raise (Bent-Over): 3 hard sets	×	×	×
Triceps Pushdown: 3 hard sets	×	×	×
Hanging Leg Raise: 3 hard sets			

NOTES:

WORKOUT 3: PULL			
EXERCISES	**SETS**		
Barbell Deadlift: Warm-up and 3 hard sets	×	×	×
Pull-Up: 3 hard sets	×	×	×
Lat Pulldown (Wide-Grip): 3 hard sets	×	×	×
Alternating Dumbbell Curl: 3 hard sets	×	×	×

NOTES:

_____

_____

_____

WORKOUT 4: LOWER BODY (LEGS AND GLUTES)			
EXERCISES	**SETS**		
Barbell Squat: Warm-up and 3 hard sets	×	×	×
Dumbbell Lunge (Reverse): 3 hard sets	×	×	×
Romanian Deadlift: 3 hard sets	×	×	×
Hip Thrust: 3 hard sets	×	×	×

NOTES:

_____

_____

_____

4-DAY ROUTINE	DELOAD	WEEK 54

WORKOUT 1: DELOAD LEGS

EXERCISES	SETS		
Barbell Squat: Warm-up and 3 sets of 5 reps with last hard set weight	×	×	×
Romanian Deadlift: 3 sets of 5 reps with last hard set weight	×	×	×
Hip Thrust: 3 sets of 5 reps with last hard set weight	×	×	×

NOTES:

WORKOUT 2: DELOAD PUSH

EXERCISES	SETS		
Barbell Bench Press: Warm-up and 3 sets of 5 reps with last hard set weight	×	×	×
Seated Dumbbell Press: 3 sets of 5 reps with last hard set weight	×	×	×
Dumbbell Bench Press: 3 sets of 5 reps with last hard set weight	×	×	×

NOTES:

WORKOUT 3: DELOAD PULL

EXERCISES	SETS		
Barbell Deadlift: Warm-up and 3 sets of 5 reps with last hard set weight	×	×	×
Barbell Row: 3 sets of 5 reps with last hard set weight	×	×	×
Lat Pulldown (Wide-Grip): 3 sets of 5 reps with last hard set weight	×	×	×

NOTES:

3-DAY ROUTINE	PHASE 6	WEEK 46

WORKOUT 1: LOWER BODY (LEGS AND GLUTES)			
EXERCISES	**SETS**		
Barbell Squat: Warm-up and 3 hard sets	✕	✕	✕
Barbell Lunge (Walking): 3 hard sets	✕	✕	✕
Leg Curl (Lying or Seated)*: 3 hard sets	✕	✕	✕
Dumbbell Step-Up: 3 hard sets	✕	✕	✕

NOTES:

WORKOUT 2: UPPER BODY AND CORE			
EXERCISES	**SETS**		
Barbell Bench Press: Warm-up and 3 hard sets	✕	✕	✕
Dip: 3 hard sets	✕	✕	✕
Dumbbell Rear Lateral Raise (Bent-Over): 3 hard sets	✕	✕	✕
Triceps Pushdown: 3 hard sets	✕	✕	✕
Weighted Sit-Up: 3 hard sets	✕	✕	✕

NOTES:

WORKOUT 3: LOWER BODY AND PULL (LEGS AND BACK)			
EXERCISES	**SETS**		
Barbell Squat: Warm-up and 3 hard sets	✕	✕	✕
Barbell Deadlift: Warm-up and 3 hard sets	✕	✕	✕
Pull-Up: 3 hard sets	✕	✕	✕
Barbell Row: 3 hard sets	✕	✕	✕
E-Z Bar Curl: 3 hard sets	✕	✕	✕

NOTES:

| 3-DAY ROUTINE | PHASE 6 | WEEK 47 |

WORKOUT 1: LOWER BODY (LEGS AND GLUTES)

EXERCISES	SETS		
Barbell Squat: Warm-up and 3 hard sets	×	×	×
Barbell Lunge (Walking): 3 hard sets	×	×	×
Leg Curl (Lying or Seated)*: 3 hard sets	×	×	×
Dumbbell Step-Up: 3 hard sets	×	×	×

NOTES:

WORKOUT 2: UPPER BODY AND CORE

EXERCISES	SETS		
Barbell Bench Press: Warm-up and 3 hard sets	×	×	×
Dip: 3 hard sets	×	×	×
Dumbbell Rear Lateral Raise (Bent-Over): 3 hard sets	×	×	×
Triceps Pushdown: 3 hard sets	×	×	×
Weighted Sit-Up: 3 hard sets	×	×	×

NOTES:

WORKOUT 3: LOWER BODY AND PULL (LEGS AND BACK)

EXERCISES	SETS		
Barbell Squat: Warm-up and 3 hard sets	×	×	×
Barbell Deadlift: Warm-up and 3 hard sets	×	×	×
Pull-Up: 3 hard sets	×	×	×
Barbell Row: 3 hard sets	×	×	×
E-Z Bar Curl: 3 hard sets	×	×	×

NOTES:

| 3-DAY ROUTINE | PHASE 6 | WEEK 48 |

WORKOUT 1: LOWER BODY (LEGS AND GLUTES)			
EXERCISES	**SETS**		
Barbell Squat: Warm-up and 3 hard sets	×	×	×
Barbell Lunge (Walking): 3 hard sets	×	×	×
Leg Curl (Lying or Seated)*: 3 hard sets	×	×	×
Dumbbell Step-Up: 3 hard sets	×	×	×

NOTES:

WORKOUT 2: UPPER BODY AND CORE			
EXERCISES	**SETS**		
Barbell Bench Press: Warm-up and 3 hard sets	×	×	×
Dip: 3 hard sets	×	×	×
Dumbbell Rear Lateral Raise (Bent-Over): 3 hard sets	×	×	×
Triceps Pushdown: 3 hard sets	×	×	×
Weighted Sit-Up: 3 hard sets	×	×	×

NOTES:

WORKOUT 3: LOWER BODY AND PULL (LEGS AND BACK)			
EXERCISES	**SETS**		
Barbell Squat: Warm-up and 3 hard sets	×	×	×
Barbell Deadlift: Warm-up and 3 hard sets	×	×	×
Pull-Up: 3 hard sets	×	×	×
Barbell Row: 3 hard sets	×	×	×
E-Z Bar Curl: 3 hard sets	×	×	×

NOTES:

| 3-DAY ROUTINE | PHASE 6 | WEEK 49 |

WORKOUT 1: LOWER BODY (LEGS AND GLUTES)

EXERCISES	SETS		
Barbell Squat: Warm-up and 3 hard sets	✕	✕	✕
Barbell Lunge (Walking): 3 hard sets	✕	✕	✕
Leg Curl (Lying or Seated)*: 3 hard sets	✕	✕	✕
Dumbbell Step-Up: 3 hard sets	✕	✕	✕

NOTES:

WORKOUT 2: UPPER BODY AND CORE

EXERCISES	SETS		
Barbell Bench Press: Warm-up and 3 hard sets	✕	✕	✕
Dip: 3 hard sets	✕	✕	✕
Dumbbell Rear Lateral Raise (Bent-Over): 3 hard sets	✕	✕	✕
Triceps Pushdown: 3 hard sets	✕	✕	✕
Weighted Sit-Up: 3 hard sets	✕	✕	✕

NOTES:

WORKOUT 3: LOWER BODY AND PULL (LEGS AND BACK)

EXERCISES	SETS		
Barbell Squat: Warm-up and 3 hard sets	✕	✕	✕
Barbell Deadlift: Warm-up and 3 hard sets	✕	✕	✕
Pull-Up: 3 hard sets	✕	✕	✕
Barbell Row: 3 hard sets	✕	✕	✕
E-Z Bar Curl: 3 hard sets	✕	✕	✕

NOTES:

3-DAY ROUTINE	PHASE 6	WEEK 50

WORKOUT 1: LOWER BODY (LEGS AND GLUTES)

EXERCISES	SETS		
Barbell Squat: Warm-up and 3 hard sets	×	×	×
Barbell Lunge (Walking): 3 hard sets	×	×	×
Leg Curl (Lying or Seated)*: 3 hard sets	×	×	×
Dumbbell Step-Up: 3 hard sets	×	×	×

NOTES:

WORKOUT 2: UPPER BODY AND CORE

EXERCISES	SETS		
Barbell Bench Press: Warm-up and 3 hard sets	×	×	×
Dip: 3 hard sets	×	×	×
Dumbbell Rear Lateral Raise (Bent-Over): 3 hard sets	×	×	×
Triceps Pushdown: 3 hard sets	×	×	×
Weighted Sit-Up: 3 hard sets	×	×	×

NOTES:

WORKOUT 3: LOWER BODY AND PULL (LEGS AND BACK)

EXERCISES	SETS		
Barbell Squat: Warm-up and 3 hard sets	×	×	×
Barbell Deadlift: Warm-up and 3 hard sets	×	×	×
Pull-Up: 3 hard sets	×	×	×
Barbell Row: 3 hard sets	×	×	×
E-Z Bar Curl: 3 hard sets	×	×	×

NOTES:

3-DAY ROUTINE	PHASE 6	WEEK 51

WORKOUT 1: LOWER BODY (LEGS AND GLUTES)

EXERCISES	SETS		
Barbell Squat: Warm-up and 3 hard sets	×	×	×
Barbell Lunge (Walking): 3 hard sets	×	×	×
Leg Curl (Lying or Seated)*: 3 hard sets	×	×	×
Dumbbell Step-Up: 3 hard sets	×	×	×

NOTES:

WORKOUT 2: UPPER BODY AND CORE

EXERCISES	SETS		
Barbell Bench Press: Warm-up and 3 hard sets	×	×	×
Dip: 3 hard sets	×	×	×
Dumbbell Rear Lateral Raise (Bent-Over): 3 hard sets	×	×	×
Triceps Pushdown: 3 hard sets	×	×	×
Weighted Sit-Up: 3 hard sets	×	×	×

NOTES:

WORKOUT 3: LOWER BODY AND PULL (LEGS AND BACK)

EXERCISES	SETS		
Barbell Squat: Warm-up and 3 hard sets	×	×	×
Barbell Deadlift: Warm-up and 3 hard sets	×	×	×
Pull-Up: 3 hard sets	×	×	×
Barbell Row: 3 hard sets	×	×	×
E-Z Bar Curl: 3 hard sets	×	×	×

NOTES:

| 3-DAY ROUTINE | PHASE 6 | WEEK 52 |

WORKOUT 1: LOWER BODY (LEGS AND GLUTES)			
EXERCISES	SETS		
Barbell Squat: Warm-up and 3 hard sets	×	×	×
Barbell Lunge (Walking): 3 hard sets	×	×	×
Leg Curl (Lying or Seated)*: 3 hard sets	×	×	×
Dumbbell Step-Up: 3 hard sets	×	×	×

NOTES:

WORKOUT 2: UPPER BODY AND CORE			
EXERCISES	SETS		
Barbell Bench Press: Warm-up and 3 hard sets	×	×	×
Dip: 3 hard sets	×	×	×
Dumbbell Rear Lateral Raise (Bent-Over): 3 hard sets	×	×	×
Triceps Pushdown: 3 hard sets	×	×	×
Weighted Sit-Up: 3 hard sets	×	×	×

NOTES:

WORKOUT 3: LOWER BODY AND PULL (LEGS AND BACK)			
EXERCISES	SETS		
Barbell Squat: Warm-up and 3 hard sets	×	×	×
Barbell Deadlift: Warm-up and 3 hard sets	×	×	×
Pull-Up: 3 hard sets	×	×	×
Barbell Row: 3 hard sets	×	×	×
E-Z Bar Curl: 3 hard sets	×	×	×

NOTES:

| 3-DAY ROUTINE | PHASE 6 | WEEK 53 |

WORKOUT 1: LOWER BODY (LEGS AND GLUTES)

EXERCISES	SETS		
Barbell Squat: Warm-up and 3 hard sets	×	×	×
Barbell Lunge (Walking): 3 hard sets	×	×	×
Leg Curl (Lying or Seated)*: 3 hard sets	×	×	×
Dumbbell Step-Up: 3 hard sets	×	×	×

NOTES:

WORKOUT 2: UPPER BODY AND CORE

EXERCISES	SETS		
Barbell Bench Press: Warm-up and 3 hard sets	×	×	×
Dip: 3 hard sets	×	×	×
Dumbbell Rear Lateral Raise (Bent-Over): 3 hard sets	×	×	×
Triceps Pushdown: 3 hard sets	×	×	×
Weighted Sit-Up: 3 hard sets	×	×	×

NOTES:

WORKOUT 3: LOWER BODY AND PULL (LEGS AND BACK)

EXERCISES	SETS		
Barbell Squat: Warm-up and 3 hard sets	×	×	×
Barbell Deadlift: Warm-up and 3 hard sets	×	×	×
Pull-Up: 3 hard sets	×	×	×
Barbell Row: 3 hard sets	×	×	×
E-Z Bar Curl: 3 hard sets	×	×	×

NOTES:

| 3-DAY ROUTINE | DELOAD | WEEK 54 |

WORKOUT 1: DELOAD LEGS

EXERCISES	SETS		
Barbell Squat: Warm-up and 3 sets of 5 reps with last hard set weight	×	×	×
Romanian Deadlift: 3 sets of 5 reps with last hard set weight	×	×	×
Hip Thrust: 3 sets of 5 reps with last hard set weight	×	×	×

NOTES:

WORKOUT 2: DELOAD PUSH

EXERCISES	SETS		
Barbell Bench Press: Warm-up and 3 sets of 5 reps with last hard set weight	×	×	×
Seated Dumbbell Press: 3 sets of 5 reps with last hard set weight	×	×	×
Dumbbell Bench Press: 3 sets of 5 reps with last hard set weight	×	×	×

NOTES:

WORKOUT 3: DELOAD PULL

EXERCISES	SETS		
Barbell Deadlift: Warm-up and 3 sets of 5 reps with last hard set weight	×	×	×
Barbell Row: 3 sets of 5 reps with last hard set weight	×	×	×
Lat Pulldown (Wide-Grip): 3 sets of 5 reps with last hard set weight	×	×	×

NOTES:

Wow.

Can you believe it's been a whole year?

You've done it. You've huffed and puffed, grinned and grimaced, sweated and sworn your way through over 100 workouts, and look at what you have to show for it.

Seriously, go look. Like what you see?

If you're not there already, you're well on your way to your best body ever, and even better, you know exactly where to go from here. You just keep eating right and training hard until you've accomplished the results you want. At this point it's just a matter of time.

As far as the specifics go, you have two clear options at this point:

You can repeat this challenge.

Many women choose to do this because they enjoy the workouts, they're happy with their results, and they've continued to make good progress.
If that's you, then there's nothing wrong with starting over from Phase 1.

You can create new workout routines.

On the other hand, many people also want to use everything they've learned and experienced to create new, highly customized workout routines to work more on specific body parts, increase the difficulty of their workouts, or simply to mix things up and do something different.

These are all perfectly valid reasons to create your own workout routines or even try other types of weightlifting programs. If you'd like some help choosing what's next, you can find a number of effective, science-based workouts to choose from on my websites.

Visit the following sites to check them out: www.muscleforlife.com/category/workouts and www.legionathletics.com/category/workouts.

For my part, I want to be there with you as you continue your journey, so if you haven't already, please do reach out to me and share your story and results so far.

The best way to reach me is email, and my address is mike@muscleforlife.com. I'd also love to feature you as a success story on my website if you're interested! If you want to see other Year One Challenge for Women success stories, you can check them out here: www.thinnerleanerstronger.com/success.

And speaking of a success story, if you haven't shared your transformation on social media yet, now's the perfect time to post about it and inspire your friends and family! Be sure to include the #thinnerleanerstronger hashtag so that other people looking for encouragement will be able to find you and follow along.

_____

Don't forget to tag me, too! Here's where we can connect:
Facebook: www.facebook.com/muscleforlifefitness
Instagram: www.instagram.com/muscleforlifefitness
YouTube: www.youtube.com/muscleforlifefitness
Twitter: www.twitter.com/muscleforlife

Oh, and don't forget to take your final measurements and pictures for your first year of *Thinner Leaner Stronger*!

First, take the following body measurements first thing in the morning, nude, after using the bathroom and before eating or drinking anything:

1. Weight

2. Waist circumference

3. OPTIONAL: Hip circumference

4. OPTIONAL: Upper-leg circumference

5. OPTIONAL: Flexed arms

Then, take flexed and unflexed pictures from the front, back, and sides, and store them in an album or folder that you can easily locate later.

Remember to show as much skin as you feel comfortable with. The more the better because it will give you the best idea of how your body is responding to the program.

Huge kudos again on finishing the program, thanks for your support, and I hope to hear from you soon!

FREE BONUS MATERIAL (VIDEOS, TOOLS, AND MORE!)

Thank you for choosing *The Year One Challenge for Women*.

I hope you found it insightful, inspiring, and practical, and I hope it helps you build that lean, sculpted, and strong body you really desire.

I want to make sure that you get as much value from this program as possible, so I've put together a number of additional free resources to help you, including:

→ All of the workouts neatly laid out and provided in several formats, including PDF, Excel, and Google Sheets.

→ Links to form demonstration videos for all *Thinner Leaner Stronger* exercises.

→ 10 *Thinner Leaner Stronger* meal plans that make losing fat and gaining lean muscle as simple as possible.

→ A Google Sheets meal planning template for simpler and easier meal planning.

→ A list of my favorite tools for getting and staying motivated and on track inside and outside of the gym.

→ My most-recommended books for building a better body and life.

→ Three interviews with thought leaders Stephen Guise, James Clear, and Mark Murphy on the topics of habit formation, goal setting and accomplishment, environment design, and more.

→ And more.

To get instant access to all of those free bonuses (plus a few additional surprise gifts), go here now:
→ www.thinnerleanerstronger.com/challengebonus

And remember: if you have any questions or run into any difficulties, just shoot me an e-mail at mike@muscleforlife.com and I'll do my best to help!

WOULD YOU DO ME A FAVOR?

Beware of monotony;
it's the mother of all the deadly sins.

—EDITH WHARTON

Thank you for reading *The Year One Challenge for Women*. I hope it has helped you look, feel, and live better than you ever have before.

I have a small favor to ask.

Would you mind taking a minute to write a blurb on Amazon about this book? I check all my reviews and love to get honest feedback. That's the real pay for my work—knowing that I'm helping people.

To leave me a review, you can . . .

1. Pull up Amazon on your web browser, search for "year one challenge women," click to the book's product page, and scroll down and click on the "Write a customer review" button.

2. Visit www.thinnerleanerstronger.com/reviewchallenge and you'll be automatically forwarded to Amazon to leave a review.

Thanks again!

DO YOU WANT ONE-ON-ONE COACHING?

Why do you want to get fit?

Sure, there's the obvious—great biceps, butts, and abs are kind of neat—but methinks it goes deeper than that.

What are the "benefits of the benefits" you're after?

Do you want to wear the clothes you really want to wear? And look fantastic when you take them off?

Do you want to be a better role model for your family and friends and promote healthy living?

Do you more intimacy in your relationships and better sex?

Do you want more confidence and self-esteem?

Do you want to be able to play with your kids without getting winded?

Do you want to jump out of bed every morning with more energy, enthusiasm, and vitality?

Or maybe you just want to stop stressing over what you see in the mirror every day and finally be comfortable in your own skin?

Whatever your reasons are, I want you to know this:

My reason for doing everything I do is to help you make your reasons a reality.

The real pay for my work isn't dollars and cents or even seeing people with leaner and more muscular bodies. It's the way I'm helping them change their lives for the better. That's priceless.

That's why I continue to write books and articles and record podcasts and videos, and why I'm always trying to push my work to the next level.

That's also why I offer a VIP one-on-one coaching service, which I'm extremely proud of.

In just a few short years, we've worked with over 450 men and women of all ages and circumstances and helped them do a lot more than lose a bunch of fat and gain a bunch of strength and muscle.

→ We've helped them skyrocket their grades and productivity.

→ We've helped them achieve promotions at work.

→ We've helped them rekindle their love lives and even save their marriages.

→ We've helped them break food, drug, and alcohol addictions.

→ We've helped them form deeper bonds with friends and family.

→ We've helped them reverse and resolve health conditions and ditch medications.

→ And so much more . . .

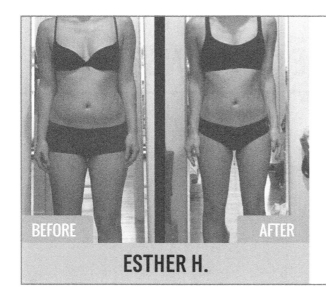

ESTHER H.

One of our clients, Esther (30), is a perfect example of what you can accomplish when experts do all the thinking for you and make your dieting and training paint-by-numbers simple.

As you can see, she dramatically improved her body composition, but she also gained a tremendous amount of strength.

For instance, when she started with us, she was deadlifting just the bar, and by the end of her 90-day coaching experience, she was close to her body weight for reps.

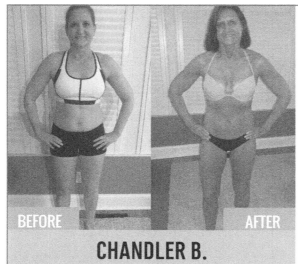

CHANDLER B.

I'm also really proud of Chandler (55), who dropped nearly 14 pounds, 6 percent body fat, and two dress sizes in just three months:

"It took a couple of weeks to kick in," she told me afterward, "but when it did, I saw progress every week, both in my body composition and the weight I was lifting."

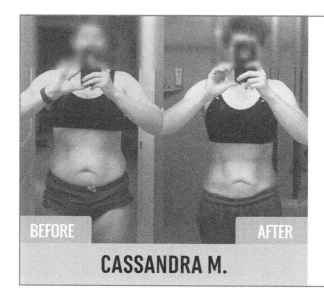

CASSANDRA M.

Cassandra (38) also killed it, reducing her waist size by five inches and weight by 25 pounds in 12 weeks. Since a picture is worth a thousand words and all that:

"I'm definitely more confident and feeling better about myself," she said afterward. "I'm feeling just better overall. I definitely have more energy and determination."

Now, what about YOU?
Do you want to make this the year
you finally get super fit?

Are you ready to transform YOUR body and life?

If so, you need to visit the following URL and schedule your free consultation call to see if my coaching service is right for you:

Go here now
→ www.muscleforlife.com/coaching

You have to hurry, though, because my coaches are always in high demand and availability is always limited.

This will NOT be a high-pressure sales call, by the way. It's a friendly chat to learn where you're at, where you've been, and where you want to go, and then determine whether the service is right for you.

You should also know that this service comes with a very simple money-back guarantee:

Either you love the experience and are thrilled with your results, or you get every penny you've paid back.

That's how much confidence I have in my team's ability to help you get great results.

So, take the first step in your journey to a fitter, happier, and healthier you.

Go to www.muscleforlife.com/coaching
and schedule your call now.

I WANT TO CHANGE THE SUPPLEMENT INDUSTRY FOR THE BETTER. WILL YOU JOIN ME?

The supplement industry is best described by Ben Kenobi's famous words:
A wretched hive of scum and villainy.

Seriously. Fake news, fake science, fake products—you can find it all in the supplement racket. It's almost funny . . . in the not so funny kind of way.

You now know that despite what supplement hucksters would have you believe, supplements don't build a great physique. Only proper diet and training does.

Furthermore, not only are supplements completely unnecessary, but most everything sitting on the shelves of your local supplement store doesn't even work. And some products can even be dangerous.

The reality is when you take a supplement, you're putting your health in the hands of complete strangers who work in an industry overflowing with cash and crooks. This is why many people have decided to stay away from supplements altogether, which is a perfectly reasonable position considering what I've just told you.

It's too bad though because not all supplements are junk. There are safe, natural supplements that can help you gain muscle, lose fat, and get healthy faster. No, they're not going to transform your body or change your life, but research shows they can give you a slight edge in your journey to a fitter and healthier you.

The problem, though, is finding high-quality products and supplement companies you can actually trust.

And so I wondered . . .

Should I "scratch my own itch" and create the supplements that I myself have always wanted? Would anyone else want them as well?

This wasn't an easy decision.

I've made my bones as an author an educator. I've sold over a million books, published over a million words of free content on my blogs, and worked with thousands of people of all ages and circumstances. And most people think that's awesome. Go me.

What would happen if I were to start selling supplements, though?

I feared that no matter how good they were or how honestly or fairly I might try to offer them, many of my readers and followers would assume the worst, reach for their pitchforks and torches, and try to run me off the internet.

And so I was on the horns of a dilemma.

On one hand, I saw an opportunity to do things very differently in the supplement space and create 100 percent natural, science-backed safe supplements that really work.

On the other hand, that would mean getting into the 20-ton-turd-salad that is the supplement industry and trying to convince people that I wasn't a lying scammer like everyone else.

And so after much deliberation and many sacrificial offerings to the gods of commerce and capitalism, I decided to go with my gut and throw my hat in the ring.

I started a supplement company called Legion Athletics (www.legionathletics.com) and wasn't sure what to expect.

Would people have enough faith in me and appreciate the products and what makes them special? Would it be a flash in the pan or would it have staying power?

Well, that was 2014 and I'm glad I made that leap of faith because Legion is now a thriving business with over 200,000 customers around the world who have left thousands and thousands of glowing reviews all over the internet.

One of the primary reasons Legion is going gangbusters is our commitment to complete transparency, from formulating to scientific research, marketing and advertising, labeling, and more.

I'm an extremely skeptical person and consumer and, quite frankly, would assume that any supplement company is guilty until proven innocent.

In other words, I've approached it from the angle of what would it take for someone like me to buy supplements from Legion? What would I need to see to be convinced?

I want to know several things:

1. I'd want to know who comes up with the formulations and what their credentials are.

   Again, we're talking about our health here, so I'd want to know a bit about the person or persons I'm trusting mine to.

2. I'd want to know exactly what's in the products.

   I'd want to know every active and inactive ingredient, and the doses of every active ingredient in particular to ensure it's not "pixie dusted" with small, ineffective amounts of ingredients or spiked with fillers or unnecessary junk.

3. I'd want to see science-based explanations of how the products are supposed to work.

   I wouldn't want flashy ads with hulking bodybuilders barking buzzwords at me.

I'd want to understand why ingredients were chosen and what they're supposed to do in the body, and I'd want to see all the published scientific research to back the claims up.

4 I'd want to see third-party proof that the products are legitimate.

I trust product labels about as much as the mainstream media, so I'd want to see certificates of analysis confirming the labels are 100 percent accurate.

5 I'd want to see what other people are saying about the products.

That means independent online reviews, reviews from verified purchasers and customers, and opinions from respected industry leaders.

If a supplement company could satisfactorily check all five of those boxes, I'd be probably willing to give them a try. Otherwise, hard pass.

If you're like me, then I think you're going to really like what I'm doing with Legion because it lives up to all of those standards, and more. Simply put, Legion outclasses everything on the market and is the yardstick by which all other supplement companies should be judged.

Visit the following URL to see for yourself:
Go here now → **wwww.legionathletics.com**

And if you like what you see and want to give my products a try, use the code TLS10 and you'll save 10 percent on your entire order.

The bottom line is I'm not just looking to build a supplement company. I'm looking to build a culture that people like you appreciate and want to be a part of.

I believe in respecting customers, telling things like they are, and delivering what I promise. I believe honesty and integrity sell better than cutting corners and relying on ridiculous advertisements and lies.

I don't just want to sell you pills and powders, I want to change the supplement industry for the better.

Will you join me?

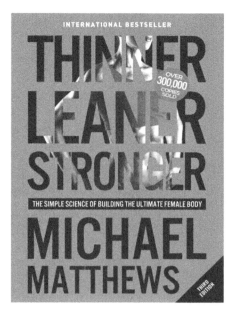

THINNER LEANER STRONGER

THE SIMPLE SCIENCE OF BUILDING
THE ULTIMATE FEMALE BODY

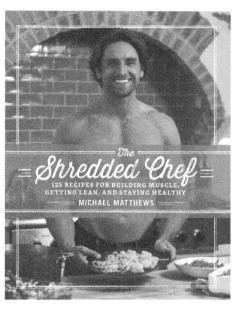

THE SHREDDED CHEF

125 RECIPES FOR BUILDING MUSCLE,
GETTING LEAN, AND STAYING HEALTHY

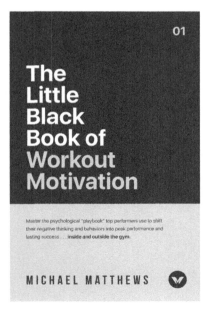

**THE LITTLE BLACK BOOK
OF WORKOUT MOTIVATION**

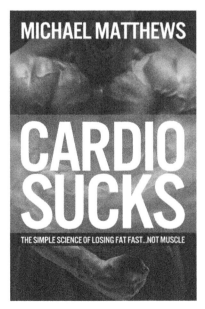

CARDIO SUCKS

THE SIMPLE SCIENCE OF LOSING
FAT FAST...NOT MUSCLE

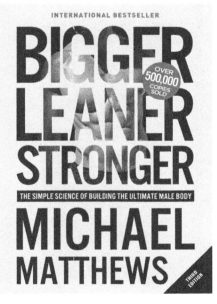

BIGGER LEANER STRONGER

THE SIMPLE SCIENCE OF BUILDING
THE ULTIMATE MALE BODY